DATE DUE

NO 24 98			
MY 3 99			
NO 17 05			

DEMCO 38-296

BEFORE BIRTH

BEFORE BIRTH

Prenatal Testing for Genetic Disease

ELENA O. NIGHTINGALE, M.D.
and MELISSA GOODMAN

HARVARD UNIVERSITY PRESS
Cambridge, Massachusetts · London, England · 1990

Library of Congress Cataloging-in-Publication Data

Nightingale, Elena O.
    Before birth: prenatal testing for genetic disease / Elena O.
Nightingale and Melissa Goodman.
        p.   cm.
    ISBN 0-674-06390-2 (alk. paper).—ISBN 0-674-06391-0 (pbk.:
alk. paper)
    1. Prenatal diagnosis—Popular works. 2. Fetus—Abnormalities—
Diagnosis. I. Goodman, Melissa, 1952–   . II. Title.
RG628.N54 1990
618.3'2042—dc20
                                                    89-19879
                                                       CIP

To my beloved family: my husband, Stuart, and
my daughters, Elizabeth and Marisa
—E.O.N.

To the memory of Fran Cunningham,
who always understood the politics
—M.G.

Contents

Foreword

by Julius B. Richmond, M.D.

In *Before Birth* the authors offer a remarkably lucid explanation of prenatal diagnosis, a subject with important ramifications for families and for prospective parents. This presentation of one aspect of the recent revolution in biology would not have been possible without the authors' rich and deep background in science and clinical medicine.

The lives of children everywhere have been transformed by medical advances in the diagnosis and treatment of acute infectious diseases. At the turn of the century the five leading causes of death among children were all infectious diseases. Today *no* infectious disease ranks among the first five causes. Because of this improvement, and the emphasis on better nutrition that has led to healthier children, researchers are able to devote their energies to other causes of childhood illness and disability—specifically, to disorders that are genetic or that result from environmental effects on the developing fetus. Concomitantly, progress in genetic and environmental research has made it possible to consider clinical applications of this newer knowledge.

The technology for prenatal diagnosis has been developing dramatically. No one set of tests can reveal all the possible unfortunate outcomes of pregnancy. The authors therefore introduce us to the whole spectrum of available technologies and the conditions that each can identify. They emphasize that al-

though there are two hundred or more diseases to which prenatal diagnosis is already applicable, tests for many more diseases will become feasible as research progresses. The nature of
the tests, their desirability or lack of desirability, and their
public health applications receive objective and comprehensive
evaluation.

Scientific progress is not without problems. Application of
the expanding knowledge in this area poses new—and sometimes difficult—choices for public health officials, parents, and
families. Economic, legal, and ethical issues arise. The authors
consider the dilemmas involved in matters such as mandatory
or voluntary screening, and the subtleties of the alternatives are
dealt with in detail. For example, in most states screening of
newborn infants is now required for phenylketonuria and hypo-
thyroidism, disorders that if not treated shortly after birth result in mental retardation.

The knowledge attained by scientific advance is never
enough for solid decision making; it only permits more informed judgment. The role of the family in making choices
about prenatal diagnostic procedures and their results is re-
viewed carefully here, as is the impact of genetic counseling,
social service programs, and support groups.

Because of the timeliness and the quality of the information
presented, this book will be of interest to professionals as well
as to the public at large. It is a model of how rapidly developing scientific knowledge and its applications can be communi-
cated to a wide audience.

Preface

Prenatal diagnosis has come a long way since the era when doctors had little more than family history available to them in their efforts to predict whether a couple was likely to have a child with a genetic disease. Today's armamentarium contains an array of tools, some fairly simple, others extremely complex. We have written this book to help prospective parents understand the new technologies for diagnosing genetic conditions prenatally so that they can make informed choices about whether to undergo these tests—and, if they do, about how to use the results.

We start by discussing what prenatal diagnosis can accomplish and who should seek it out. Several of the tests are explained, as well as the conditions they screen for. Because prospective parents frequently want to know how a specific genetic disease would affect their offspring and their family life, we have described five of these disorders in some detail.

The potential drain on the family, financially and emotionally, when a child is born with one of these diseases is enormous; inevitably the question arises of whether to terminate the pregnancy before birth. Abortion is an extremely sensitive issue, and we want to make our position clear. We respect people's objections to abortion, whether for religious, for philosophical, or for other reasons. Nonetheless, we believe that prospective parents should have the right to decide for themselves, without coercion or political pressure, whether they wish to continue or interrupt a pregnancy.

We hope that by the time you have finished this book you will better understand why genetic diseases occur, what can be done to diagnose them before birth, and how to make informed choices about the use of prenatal diagnosis. If you need more information or help in dealing with a specific condition, we have included an appendix that lists some resources.

Many people have had a role in this project. Howard Boyer of Harvard University Press had the foresight to predict not only that the two of us would work well together but that we would enjoy our collaboration. We are grateful for the steadfast support and contributions of Vivian Wheeler, also of Harvard University Press. Eve Nichols and Judith Weinblatt offered us loan privileges at their voluminous libraries and raised many provocative issues. They, along with Revella Levin and innumerable others, listened patiently during the trials and tribulations of writing this book.

E.O.N.

M.G.

BEFORE BIRTH

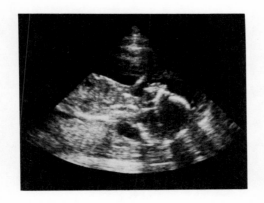

Introduction

Amy Ross-Chamberlin and Carl Chamberlin had anticipated the birth of their first child with great joy and high hopes for the future. At age twenty-eight, Amy, a computer programmer, was established in her job and planned to take a three-month leave of absence when the baby was born. Carl, at twenty-nine, enjoyed his work as a newspaper editor and looked forward to the challenges of parenting. Within three months of deciding that they were ready to start their family, Amy became pregnant. Apart from the usual morning sickness, Amy felt fine throughout her pregnancy and continued to work until her ninth month. Ten days prior to her due date, she went into labor.

Although the labor lasted a little longer than expected, Carl stayed with Amy to coach her and support her through natural childbirth. He watched in awe as their much-wanted son slid into the obstetrician's waiting hands. Then, abruptly, joy gave way to tragedy. The doctor saw immediately that the child was not well. His breathing was shallow. His tongue was a little larger than normal. He had short, stubby fingers and a crease across his palms. Most tellingly, he was quite limp and had a fold of skin around his eyes that gave him an abnormal appearance.

Although the doctor strongly suspected Down syndrome, a genetic condition characterized by mental retardation and a shortened life span, he did not wish to alarm Carl and Amy without proof that his suspicions were true. Yet the look on his face told Carl immediately that something was wrong. In response to Carl's insistent questions, the physician hedged and said that the baby was not breathing as vigorously as he should be and would need a little extra care.

The obstetrician called in a pediatrician to evaluate the infant. She performed a thorough physical examination and determined that the child faced no immediate danger. She took a blood sample to the laboratory, which in a few days sent back a preliminary positive report. Two weeks later the final report confirmed that baby Ethan had Down syndrome.

The couple felt as if their world had come to an end. Instead of a healthy baby, they were taking home a child who would probably be dependent on them or on others for the rest of his life. The pediatrician told them that at this early stage no one could predict how disabled their son would be. She was unable to say if he would be so profoundly retarded that he would never learn to talk, walk, or attend to his basic needs. Or if he would be one of those individuals with Down syndrome who attains the skills of a first or second grader (able to dress himself, feed himself, tend to his basic hygiene, learn to read, perform simple arithmetic) and eventually is capable of working in a sheltered situation.

Sadly, the pediatrician told Carl and Amy to bring Ethan in for routine checkups and to watch for early signs of infection, to which children with Down syndrome are particularly susceptible. She encouraged them to enroll the child in an infant-stimulation program to maximize his potential. And she suggested that after a few months they seek genetic counseling.

Suddenly Carl and Amy found themselves facing more questions than answers: How did this happen? Why didn't the doctor warn us? Couldn't he have tested the child for this condition before he was born? What should we do with our son?

Should we raise him ourselves? Or should we put him up for adoption by a couple who know they want a handicapped child? And, perhaps most frightening of all, what will happen if we decide to have another child—will that child be affected too?

The Chamberlins are not alone in their anguish and uncertainty. Each year over 100,000 infants in the United States are born with a genetic disease. Down syndrome is one of the five most common, potentially affecting 1 in every 1,000 births. Other common genetic afflictions are sickle cell disease, which affects about 1 in 400 children born to African-Americans; neural tube defects, which affect 1 in 800 infants; cystic fibrosis, which affects about 1 in 1,600 Caucasians; and Tay-Sachs disease, which potentially affects 1 in 3,600 Americans of Eastern European Jewish ancestry.

One way of lessening the incidence of birth defects, and of allowing couples at risk for giving birth to children with genetic afflictions the greatest chance of having healthy children, is prenatal screening. The term refers to the procedure of identifying *before a fetus is born* whether or not it has a serious congenital or genetic disorder. In some cases the process begins even before the couple decide to have a child. Consider, for example, a Jewish couple of Eastern European ancestry who want to have a child but know that because of their heritage they have a higher than usual risk of producing a child with Tay-Sachs disease, a devastating condition from which children die in their early years. The couple can have themselves tested to see if they carry the gene for this condition. If both do have the gene, each of their children will have a 1-in-4 chance of developing Tay-Sachs disease. Armed with this knowledge, the prospective parents are better equipped to make the necessary choices about how to proceed.

For most genetic diseases the technology does not yet exist

to determine before conception how likely it is that a particular couple will have an affected child. But by the mid-1970s doctors had learned how to take samples of the amniotic fluid that cushions the fetus in the womb. By analyzing its contents, they can determine whether the fetus has any one of an array of genetic conditions. Ever-evolving sampling techniques and sophisticated tests permit important determinations about the condition of the fetus earlier and earlier in the pregnancy.

A number of factors signal that a couple should consider prenatal screening. The most common is that the age of the prospective mother is thirty-five or more. Because the risk of bearing a child with a chromosomal anomaly such as Down syndrome increases substantially after this time, the mother is often advised to undergo testing to determine the status of the fetus. Likewise, a woman with a family history of chromosomal abnormalities, or one who has already given birth to a child with a chromosomal anomaly, is a good candidate for prenatal screening.

A couple who have given birth to at least one child with a condition known to have a genetic component may also want to consider prenatal screening. Examples of these conditions include spina bifida, a failure of normal closure of the spinal column; alpha-1-antitrypsin deficiency, which may destroy the liver and the lungs; the crippling and fatal Duchenne's muscular dystrophy; and the blood-clotting disorders hemophilia A and B. More than two hundred conditions can be diagnosed prenatally, and the diagnostic technology is changing so fast that tests that were unavailable when an earlier child was born may today be at hand.

People who belong to an ethnic group known to be associated with certain recessively inherited genetic conditions (see Chapter 1) may wish to have themselves tested to see if they carry a gene for this condition. Even if they are not affected themselves, if a child they conceive inherits a gene for the condition from each parent, he or she may develop the condition. As we have seen, Tay-Sachs is an example of this type of genetic disease; so are blood disorders called thalassemias, which for the most part affect people of Mediterranean ancestry.

A woman who has had two unexplained miscarriages or a child who was stillborn for unknown reasons may also find prenatal screening helpful.

Finally, anyone with a family member who has any undiagnosed abnormalities, including mental retardation, may seek prenatal screening.

The first step is to obtain genetic counseling. The family physician, obstetrician, internist, or pediatrician can usually provide basic information about genetic diseases and make a referral where appropriate. Until the mid-1970s one could obtain genetic services only in major academic medical centers, and then only if one could pay for them or was willing to participate in a research program. In 1976 the National Genetic Diseases Act initiated federal funding of genetic service programs, greatly expanding their availability. Today most medical centers have genetics units that offer diagnostic treatment and counseling services for the most common inherited disorders. Most such services are covered, at least in part, by health insurance programs such as Blue Cross and Blue Shield. Representatives from these companies can explain in detail what is included in and excluded from their benefit package.

The aim of genetic counseling is to inform patients and their families about the nature of a particular genetic disorder and the risk of its occurrence in family members. The genetic counselor can be either a medical doctor with specialized training in diagnosing and treating genetic disorders, or a counselor who works with a team of experts that includes a physician specialized in genetic disorders.

A genetic workup begins by establishing a definitive diagnosis. The counselor constructs a diagram of the blood relationships and medical histories within the family; this is referred to as a pedigree. Although, as in Carl and Amy's case, a genetic disease can occur in a family with no background of such a disease, outlining a family history in this way can uncover the previously unrecognized relevance of other medical problems. In some instances the genetics team may ask to assess other family members via physical examination and laboratory tests. Or the team may decide, if permission is granted, to obtain medical records or autopsy reports of affected relatives, to confirm a suspected diagnosis.

Once a definitive diagnosis has been reached, genetic counselors outline for the family what is known about the condition. They often understand what causes it, what the life course of a child with the disease is likely to be, and how the affliction can best be treated and managed. They can describe how it is inherited and explain how parents who are not sick themselves can pass a gene on to their children, who can become sick. The genetic counselor can also explain apparent enigmas such as the fact that only boys, and not their sisters, develop certain conditions. Medical science does not have an answer for every question, though. Sometimes parents never find out why their child was stricken. And, as in Ethan's case, the long-term outlook will become apparent only as time passes.

The vast majority of those who undergo prenatal diagnosis receive good news: for 95 percent of prospective parents, testing indicates that the fetus is free of the suspected condition. The remaining 5 percent face a painful personal decision; for, with few exceptions, at this time genetic diseases cannot be treated. The decision must be made in a social arena in which extremists on the one side believe that abortion should again be illegal and extremists on the other side believe that women who knowingly give birth to children with genetic diseases should be found legally liable.

The same technological developments that enable physicians to provide patients with very useful information and ultimately prevent great suffering also present ethical and legal quandaries. Physicians carrying out prenatal assessments sometimes come across information they have neither sought nor want. A doctor who finds, for example, that the fetus has a small chromosomal abnormality of unknown meaning must then decide what to tell the couple.

And prenatal screening is not a fail-safe process. The potential for error is inherent in the tests, or human error may occur, leading some people to believe that a condition is not present when it actually is, on the one hand, and leading people to believe that it is present when in fact it is not. Furthermore, prenatal screening is specific only for the disease in question. Prenatal screening for sickle cell disease, for example, may indicate that a child is free of that affliction, but the same child may have some other genetic or nongenetic problem that goes undetected. Screening for one disease is no guarantee of a perfect baby: 3 to 5 percent of newborns have a serious defect of some sort.

In addition, a physician will not test for a condition unless he or she believes the fetus to be at sufficient risk for that condition. Although Down syndrome does occur in pregnancies of young women, Carl and Amy's doctor, examining healthy prospective parents in their late twenties, saw no reason to put Amy through the risk and expense of testing for Down syndrome. Yet physicians who fail to stay current with the changing capabilities of prenatal diagnostic technology and fail to treat patients according to the standards of their peers can be found guilty of malpractice.

The new technologies also have broader ethical and legal implications that society as a whole must ponder. For example, it is now possible early in pregnancy to identify sickle cell disease, a crippling condition that affects people of African ancestry. Yet many poor women, especially African-American women, tend not to obtain prenatal care of any type until it is too late for prenatal testing. This issue will become even more urgent as medical advances close the gap between the present 24-week limit on legal abortions and the ability to save babies born after shorter gestation periods. At present, however, survival outside the womb of fetuses younger than 22 to 23 weeks seems unlikely.

Another impending societal issue is the incorporation of prenatal screening into the health care system. As one instance, scientists expect in the near future to perfect a test that will permit mass screening for cystic fibrosis. This life-threatening disease, which affects the lungs and digestive system, is the most common genetic disorder in Caucasians. If all white couples were to seek screening for cystic fibrosis, they would overwhelm the current system. Society must decide who is to receive prenatal screening services, and who is to pay for them.

Once the genetic counselor has assembled all the available information, he or she can help the couple assess the options for dealing with the situation in a manner consonant with their goals, values, resources, and religious beliefs. But the parents must decide for themselves whether or not to risk having a child with a genetic disease. They must decide what to do if they find that their pregnancy is affected by a devastating illness. They must weigh having an abortion against the medical services an afflicted child would require at birth and in the years to come. The genetic counselor can help explore possibilities for child care and for financial help and other resources, but the couple alone must determine if they as a family can cope with the situation—emotionally, medically, and financially.

Many couples find it helpful to seek supplemental guidance from a pastoral counselor, a mental health professional, or a specific support group in answering these and the many other questions and concerns they face.

Another significant job of the genetic counselor is to help inform prospective parents about the risk that a particular genetic disease will occur in future pregnancies. Environmental factors may contribute to the development of birth defects, and the counselor will want to explore possible exposures to harmful substances. Parents can be told what tests are available for identifying the genetic disease in question. Every test has both benefits and limitations; some involve risk to the mother or child.

Depending on the findings, the couple may choose to undergo testing of each pregnancy and consider aborting any affected fetus. They may use artificial insemination or donation of an egg by a person known not to have a gene for the disease in question. This noncarrier can be artificially inseminated by the carrier's husband; either the noncarrier can take the pregnancy to term herself or the embryo can be transferred to the carrier's uterus. In vitro fertilization is another possibility. These reproductive options are difficult, expensive, and of variable success. The couple may decide to forgo bearing their own children and try instead to adopt. Or, happily, they may learn from the tests that their potential children are not at risk and so augment their family with peace of mind.

The information the genetic counselor provides can often seem overwhelmingly complicated. Parents may need to hear it several times in different ways before they can understand and use the data. Our purpose in writing this book is to assist those who are trying to sort out their options.

We have already suggested what prenatal diagnosis can accomplish and who should seek it out. In Chapter 1 we review the process of inheritance down to the molecular level. Some readers may not be interested in this much detail, but we include it for those who wish to understand how the process can go awry and end up creating an individual with a genetic disease. In Chapter 2 we turn to the practical matter of what tests are available for diagnosing genetic diseases prenatally. We indicate how the tests are performed, what they can reveal, and what their limitations and hazards are.

When asked if they wish to undergo a test for a particular condition, parents often want to know how the condition would affect their offspring and their families. For this reason we explain in Chapter 3 how five common genetic diseases might affect a family's life course. In the next two chapters we place the capabilities of the new technologies in their ethical and legal contexts and articulate the dilemmas that sometimes must be faced. In the Conclusion we return to Amy and Carl, with whom we began our story, and describe how they came to grips, at least temporarily, with their difficult situation.

CHAPTER 1

The Mechanisms of Inheritance

The "stuff that genes are made of" is deoxyribonucleic acid, or DNA. It is the material responsible for transmitting characteristics from parent to child. DNA molecules are very long spirals, packaged neatly in chromosomes. Found in every body cell, chromosomes are small rods visible under the microscope. They are the bearers of heredity. This chapter describes the role of chromosomes, genes, and DNA in passing our genetic heritage from generation to generation.

CHROMOSOMES

The potential for new human life begins at conception—the moment sperm meets egg. At this instant the genetic lottery is over and the genetic characteristics of the person-to-be are determined. Every normal sperm and every normal egg, both of which are referred to as gametes, carry hereditary material in 23 densely packed, rod-shaped bundles called chromosomes. The chromosomes arrive in the gametes at the end of an ordered process of replication and distribution, a precise dance of pairing and separation called meiosis or reduction division. Every human cell except the egg and sperm has 46 chromosomes. Reduction division in gametes permits the new individual to have 46 chromosomes just like each parent. If this pairing and separation did not take place, each generation would have twice the chromosomes of the one before. The fetus that eventually develops from the union of sperm and egg thus acquires half its hereditary material from its father and half from its mother, in the form of 23 pairs of chromosomes.

By convention, scientists number chromosomal pairs roughly in order of decreasing size. Chromosomal pairs 1 through 22 are called autosomes; each member of a pair looks just like its partner and differs in genetic content and appearance from all the other pairs. The twenty-third chromosomes are called the sex chromosomes, since their content determines whether the fetus is male or female. A normal egg always carries an X sex chromosome. A normal sperm can carry either an X or a Y. Thus, a fetus always inherits an X chromosome from its mother. If it also inherits an X from its father, it will be a female; if it inherits a Y from its father, it will be a male. In other words, only the father's genetic contribution determines whether the baby will be a boy or a girl.

Much can be learned by studying the chromosomal makeup of the individual even before birth, by means of the procedures to be described in the next chapter. In amniocentesis the physician removes a sample of amniotic fluid, the liquid that surrounds the fetus. This fluid contains cells called fibroblasts, shed by the fetus, that reveal its genetic makeup. Fetal cells can also be obtained for analysis by chorionic villus sampling. Or the doctor can take a sample of blood or skin from a newborn or its parents to study their chromosomes. (It is possible to take a blood sample from the fetus, but the procedure is rather risky. A new method, called percutaneous umbilical blood sampling, that removes blood from the umbilical cord seems safer.)

In a type of study called a karyotype, the white blood cells, or skin fibroblasts, can be made to grow in the laboratory; their chromosomes are subsequently stained and examined under a microscope. To construct a karyotype, the researcher photographically "captures" the chromosomes in suspended anima-tion during cell division, then magnifies the photographs. In a cut-and-paste exercise, he or she cuts the chromosomes out of the photograph, lines them up in descending order of size by pairs, and examines them carefully for changes in shape or arrangement.

Sometimes in the process of preparing the karyotype, the geneticist will spot one or more extra chromosomes, or an extra or missing piece of chromosomal material. Ethan, for example, had three chromosomes instead of two in the twenty-first position (Figure 1). This chromosomal makeup, referred to as trisomy 21, is the hallmark of Down syndrome, which affects about 1 in 1,000 infants born alive in the United States. It is the most common form of trisomy, but a child can inherit an extra one of any chromosome. In fact, some infants inherit one chromosome less. Pieces of chromosomes can also get lost within the cell or become attached to the wrong chromosome.

Many specialists believe that a large percentage of the embryos that abort naturally during the first few weeks of pregnancy are afflicted with devastating chromosomal defects so severe as to be incompatible with life. A smaller number are spontaneously aborted later in pregnancy, and a still smaller number of babies with severe chromosomal defects die in the early months of life.

From studying the karyotype, and without even meeting the patient, the technician will know immediately whether the number, shape, and size of the whole set of chromosomes is normal or not and whether the fetus is male or female, since every normal male has an XY chromosomal pair in the twenty-third position and every normal female has two XX chromosomes in that position. Because of errors that occur when the gametes are formed, however, there are some variations from these norms. Approximately 1 girl in 1,500 born alive, for example, inherits only a single X chromosome. Girls with this

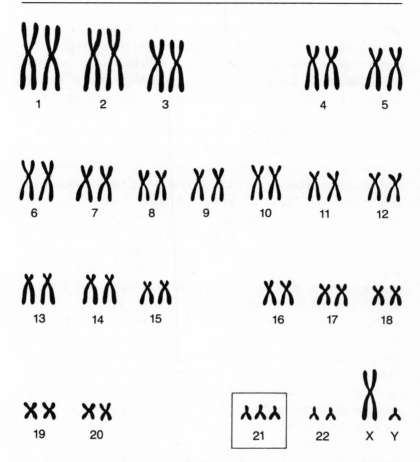

Figure 1. The karyotype of a boy with Down syndrome has an extra chromosome number 21, so that there are three instead of the normal two. This condition most often results from an incomplete separation of the chromosomes when the egg is formed in the ovary. The chromosomes can be stained to reveal patterns of bands that aid in identification. Adapted from National Institute of General Medical Sciences, *The New Human Genetics,* NIH Publication 84-662, September 1984, p. 12.

condition usually have normal intelligence but are shorter than average, usually fail to menstruate and ovulate as they mature, and are sterile. About 1 girl in 1,000 inherits three X chromosomes. These girls, as they mature, are usually normal in appearance and are fertile.

Males too can inherit abnormal sex chromosomes. Some are born with two X chromosomes and a Y chromosome. Men with this constitution, called Klinefelter syndrome, look fairly normal but are tall, have small testicles, and are usually sterile; some are also mentally retarded. Roughly 1 boy in 1,000 born alive has Klinefelter syndrome, making it about as common as Down syndrome. At least one X chromosome is needed to sustain life. When a Y chromosome is present, regardless of the number of X chromosomes, the individual looks masculine. When two Y chromosomes are present, the baby will develop into a rather tall boy who may otherwise be quite normal.

GENES

A detailed look at the structure of chromosomes reveals that they are laden with an astonishing number of genes, the basic units of heredity. Each of us carries a total of about 100,000 genes on our chromosomes. The nature of a person's genes determines the traits inherited—for example, eye color and blood type.

Scientists have identified about 4,000 genetic disorders that are caused by a flaw in one gene. At first it may be hard to imagine how a single defective gene could debilitate the entire body or even extinguish life. Consider, though, that genes contain the information that cells use to construct protein molecules. These proteins then direct the essential chemical or metabolic processes in the cell. The proteins can be either enzymes, which regulate the speed of biochemical processes, or building blocks, which the cells use for complex construction processes. If a specific enzyme is defective or absent, this deficiency disturbs a specific biochemical reaction and every subsequent reaction dependent on it.

Eve K. Nichols has described this process in *Human Gene Therapy* (Cambridge, Massachusetts: Harvard University Press, 1988). Except for blood disorders, she notes, most genetic disorders that result in viable offspring are caused by faulty enzymes. For example, in the single-gene disorder phenylketonuria (PKU), the enzyme phenylalanine hydroxylase is deficient. Under normal conditions this enzyme converts the amino acid phenylalanine into tyrosine. When the enzyme cannot do its job, phenylalanine accumulates in the body, interfering with the development of brain cells and causing mental retardation.

In other types of metabolic conditions, inherited enzyme deficiencies disrupt the orderly construction and reconstruction of essential chemical compounds that usually take place in the cells. In the normal person large molecules are broken down and their pieces reused or discarded. But children with Tay-Sachs disease, for example, cannot make the enzyme hexosaminidase A. Therefore, complex molecules derived from the central nervous system and usually broken down by this enzyme accumulate in the nerve cells of the brain and cause blindness, paralysis, and death during early childhood.

Modes of Transmission

Some single-gene disorders are autosomal dominant, some are autosomal recessive, and some are X linked or sex linked; each type is transmitted differently. As their names imply, the first two means of transmission involve genes on the nonsex (autosomal) chromosomes. Since the fetus receives half its genetic makeup from its mother and half from its father, it inherits one gene from each parent for each autosomally transmitted trait.

To develop an autosomal-dominant disease, an individual need inherit only a single faulty gene for that disease from one of the two parents. That parent almost always has some manifestation of the disease. The effect of this gene is so powerful that it "dominates" its normal counterpart. The offspring of an afflicted couple therefore faces a 50 percent chance of inheriting the faulty gene—and the disorder—from the affected parent. Occasionally a person develops a dominantly inherited condition without a family history of it because of spontaneous change or mutation of the gene to the dominant form. The children of this individual have a 50 percent chance of inheriting the condition, but the affected person's brothers and sisters are almost always normal because a mutation usually occurs only in one egg or sperm—the one that gave rise to the affected individual.

One extremely distressing autosomal-dominant disorder is Huntington's disease, a degenerative neurological condition that usually does not appear until adulthood. A test has become available that can tell people who have an affected parent but are still normal themselves whether or not they carry the gene for this disease.

Another autosomal-dominant condition is familial hypercholesterolemia, in which the body produces as much as five times the normal amount of cholesterol. Even children with this condition can develop coronary artery disease and have heart attacks.

To develop an autosomal-recessive condition, on the other hand, a child must inherit a pair of mutant genes, one from each parent. The parents, generally unaffected by the disorder, both carry a defective gene for the condition but are protected against developing it because they also have a normal gene for that trait that can compensate for the defective one. People with one gene for a recessive disease are referred to as carriers. Each of the children of two carriers has a 25 percent chance of inheriting a double dose of the defective gene and therefore the genetic defect. Each also has a 25 percent chance of inheriting two normal genes and a 50 percent chance of being a carrier like the parents. Common autosomal-recessive disorders are sickle cell disease, cystic fibrosis, and Tay-Sachs disease, all of which are described in Chapter 3.

Finally, the X-linked, or sex-linked, disorders are so named because the faulty gene lies on the X, or sex, chromosome. Sex-linked disorders affect males and females differently, because females have two X chromosomes and males have only one. A disorder of blood clotting leading to uncontrolled bleeding in males, hemophilia A, is the most common sex-linked condition.

In a typical scenario the father has normal chromosomes and is normal himself. The mother, who has the defective (recessive) gene on one of her two X chromosomes, does not develop the disease because her normal X chromosome compensates for the defect on the other. Each of her children has a 50 percent chance of inheriting the abnormal gene on an X chromosome, but only her sons develop the disease because the Y chromosome inherited from the father cannot counteract the faulty gene on the X chromosome (the X and Y chromosomes do not have matching genes). Daughters who inherit the defective gene are usually free of the condition, because they, like their mother, have the compensating normal gene. And, like her, they are carriers and can pass the gene on to their own sons. Thus, X-linked disorders are passed from normal mothers to their sons and never from fathers to sons.

Chance and Risk

The "chance" of developing a genetic condition can be a difficult concept to grasp. To say that a fetus has a 1-in-4 chance of developing cystic fibrosis does not mean that one of four members of a particular family will actually develop the condition; the risk figure applies to the population at large. Nor does it mean that if a couple has one child with this condition, the next three will be free of it. The risk of 1 in 4, or 25 percent, applies to each pregnancy individually.

In many ways the notion of chance lies at the heart of the development of inherited disease. Chance, among other things, determines which man will come together with which woman to have a child. Chance, among other things, determines which sperm will unite with which egg, and which abnormal genes will be present on the chromosomes of these gametes. Because of these chance encounters, about 3 or 4 percent of all babies born have a serious genetic disease or birth defect that could not have been predicted or tested for. Every normal person probably carries somewhere on his or her chromosomes several abnormal genes that if present in double dose would cause a major problem or death.

In order to comprehend how easy it is for nature to make a mistake during the hereditary process and thus give rise to genetic disease, one must understand the complex molecule that is the central player in the drama of heredity.

DNA

We have said that the double-helical molecule DNA is the stuff of which genes are made. Within its two long, twisted strands DNA harbors in coded form the material that allows cells to function. Its basic subunits are the nucleotides, each of which consists of one sugar molecule, one phosphate group, and one of four bases—adenine, thymine, cytosine, or guanine. To use Maya Pines's image in *The New Human Genetics*, these nucleotides line up like the two sides of a zipper: the phosphate and sugar form the outer ribbon, or backbone of the helices, and the bases act like the zipper's interlocking teeth (Figure 2).

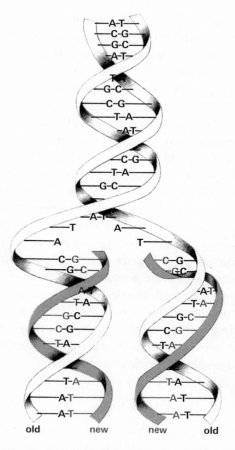

Figure 2. To reproduce itself, the DNA double helix uncoils, the strands separate, and each strand forms a template for its complement, a mirror image of itself. The "rungs" of the DNA helical ladder are made of base pairs, A always pairs with T, and C with G. The new DNA double helices are identical to the parent. A = adenine, T = thymine, C = cytosine, G = guanine. From Arthur Kornberg, *For the Love of Enzymes* (Cambridge, Mass.: Harvard University Press, 1989), p. 224.

The bases do not stay locked together all the time, however. When cells prepare to divide, the two strands of the DNA helix separate, and each one acts as a template for the creation of its mirror image. This duplication provides each new cell with the same genetic data as the original cell from which it was formed. An intermediary called ribonucleic acid, or RNA, transmits the instructions contained in the DNA to "manufacturing plants" within the cell. RNA is similar to DNA except that its sugar ribose contains more oxygen than deoxyribose, DNA's sugar. RNA is also single stranded rather than double stranded like DNA and uses the base uracil instead of thymine.

Once the RNA supplies the coded material to the manufacturing plants, the cell begins to decipher the genetic code and build the all-important proteins that the cell needs to survive. The letters of the genetic code are the different nucleotide bases. Every multiple of three nucleotide bases is referred to as a codon; every triplet either codes for a specific amino acid or signals the cell to start or stop stringing amino acids together.

Amino acids are the building blocks of proteins, and each amino acid has its own unique code. Thus, if the cell's machinery first encounters a cytosine base, then an adenine base, then another cytosine base, the instructions are to add histidine to the growing string of amino acids. There are 20 essential amino acids in all: alanine, arginine, asparagine, aspartic acid, cysteine, glutamic acid, glutamine, glycine, histidine, isoleucine, leucine, lysine, methionine, phenylalanine, proline, serine, threonine, tryptophan, tyrosine, and valine.

The order in which a cell strings together its amino acids may seem relatively unimportant. But consider the case of sickle cell anemia. Patients with this hereditary condition have chronic anemia and painful episodes caused by obstruction of their small blood vessels. The whole debilitating disorder results from the misplacement of a single nucleotide base in the affected person's DNA. This error affects the amino acid sequence of the hemoglobin, or oxygen-carrying protein. Normal hemoglobin has within it the following sequence of amino acids: valine, histidine, leucine, threonine, proline, glutamic acid, and another glutamic acid. The hemoglobin of a patient with sickle cell anemia, however, contains a second valine instead of the first glutamic acid. When reading the individual's DNA sequence, the cell's machinery has encountered guanine, thymine, guanine and therefore makes valine, whereas under normal circumstances the acids encountered are guanine, adenine, guanine, which cause the cell to make glutamic acid.

WHAT CAUSES BIRTH DEFECTS?

Every human cell contains about 6 feet of DNA, or 6 billion base pairs, coiled and packed into its 46 chromosomes. Given the extraordinary amount of material to be passed from parent to child, it is no wonder that errors occur. In addition to inexplicable birth defects, however, a number of external or environmental factors, known as teratogens, can cause damage that often is difficult to distinguish from that resulting from inherited birth defects. The developing fetus is especially vulnerable during its first two months, when its basic organ systems are forming. Damage during this time can cause abnormalities in many systems at once—the heart, the central nervous system, the gastrointestinal tract, and the kidneys, for example.

One of the best-known teratogens is thalidomide. This tranquilizer was commonly prescribed in Europe in the 1960s, and many women who used it during their pregnancies bore infants with shortened or missing limbs. Babies in the United States were spared the effects of this powerful drug, since the Food and Drug Administration did not approve its use here after learning of its tragic consequences overseas.

The genetic counselor will usually explore the possibility that the fetus was exposed to a teratogen to help advise a parent about the risks that might be associated with future pregnancies. The most common agents that can harm a fetus are alcohol, cigarettes, drugs—especially cocaine (crack) and heroin—used during pregnancy, the mother's medical condition, and viruses or other infectious agents. Alcohol has been shown to cause serious malformations and mental retardation. It reaches the placenta easily, and therefore the baby is affected by whatever the mother drinks. Although the effects of an occasional drink are not known, there is no proof that alcohol even in small amounts is safe for the baby. Cigarette smoking can cause the baby to die or to be born too small for a healthy start in life and can also cause other problems. Both alcohol and cigarettes should be totally avoided during pregnancy, as should all recreational drugs.

A number of prescribed medications, when taken by a pregnant woman, are thought to be associated with birth defects. The connection is difficult to prove; for obvious ethical reasons physicians do not want to expose a developing fetus to a potentially harmful substance. To determine the safety of a medication, they must rely on animal tests that are designed to resemble the human situation as closely as possible. If the drug causes birth defects in animals, scientists urge caution in human usage. The thalidomide tragedy demonstrates the limitations of this process: tests on rats and mice did not reveal thalidomide's teratogenicity. Thalidomide *is* a teratogen in rabbits, which unfortunately were not chosen as the animal model.

Despite these limitations, experience with some drugs shows that they are associated with birth defects frequently enough that pregnant women should avoid taking them unless a doctor deems them necessary. Some of these substances are listed below by generic name; the brand names under which they are sold are given in parentheses:

Antibiotics, such as tetracycline and streptomycin
Antiseizure medications, such as phenytoin (Dilantin) and others
The anticoagulant warfarin (Coumadin, Panwarfin, Sofarin)
Hormones, such as diethylstilbestrol and androgens
Most drugs used to treat cancer
Isotretinoin (Accutane) used in cases of severe cystic acne
Lithium, utilized to treat manic, or bipolar, depression

Because the most harm is done in the first six to eight weeks of development and pregnancy is often not diagnosed until that time or later, all women who think they might be pregnant should take the above precautions. In general, they are well advised to avoid *all* over-the-counter or prescription medications unless absolutely necessary.

Sometimes a pregnant woman can have an infection that generates so few symptoms that she does not even know she has it. Yet it can devastate the fetus. The best-known example is rubella, or German measles, which can cause deafness, heart defects, and blindness in the child. Therefore, parents should be sure that their daughters are immunized against German measles. If a young woman contemplating pregnancy is uncertain about whether she has been immunized or has had rubella, she should ask her doctor to order a test of her blood to check the antibody levels for immunity to the disease. If necessary, she can then be immunized before she becomes pregnant.

Sexually transmitted diseases can also seriously injure the developing child. Genital herpes simplex can cause severe brain damage to a baby if the affected mother has a flare-up at the time of delivery. Gonorrhea can cause eye infection and blindness if the baby is not treated immediately after birth.

And a child who acquires syphilis from its mother can develop bone malformations and other defects.

Certain medical conditions in the mother also affect the likelihood that her offspring will have birth defects. A woman with diabetes, for example, is three to four times more likely to have a child with birth defects than the average woman. The risk can be kept to a minimum by ensuring tight control of the diabetes before she becomes pregnant and throughout the pregnancy.

The same principle applies to women with phenylketonuria. With strict adherence to phenylalanine-restricted diets during the first ten years of life, and the availability of supplements that supply other essential nutrients, many women with this hereditary condition now have normal intelligence and live to childbearing age. They have high levels of phenylalanine in their blood, but it no longer affects them directly because it is only harmful during the early years when the brain is developing rapidly. The high levels of phenylalanine in the mother's blood do, however, act as a potent toxin to the developing fetus and cause mental retardation. One proposed solution is to start women with PKU on a low-phenylalanine diet before conception and have them maintain that diet throughout pregnancy. Another technically possible alternative, although highly complex emotionally and mentioned only for completeness, is for the woman and her husband to use in vitro fertilization and have the embryo transferred to the womb of a woman who does not have PKU, thereby providing the baby with a healthy surrogate environment.

A frequent cause of concern is exposure to radiation. If x-ray studies are needed, it should be determined if the woman is pregnant. If she needs, say, a single chest x-ray or an x-ray to appraise a broken arm, she is not likely to jeopardize her baby. But multiple exposures, as in a series of x-rays to evaluate an intestinal disorder, can cause problems. Precautions such as the use of a lead shield should be taken to protect the fetus if x-ray assessment is deemed essential.

Knowledge of the basic mechanisms of inheritance and the nature of the genetic material will help in understanding the procedures that doctors use in prenatal screening, as well as the limitations of the information obtained. As will become evident, prenatal screening offers many prospective parents who are at risk of having children with serious conditions the possibility of having a normal child.

CHAPTER 2

Tests and Procedures

The tests used in prenatal screening are designed to detect genetic diseases or defects in the embryo or fetus while it is still in the mother's womb. On rare occasions, the condition found can be treated prenatally; more often, the parents are enabled to better prepare for the birth of an affected child. Prenatal screening also leaves open the option of interrupting the pregnancy when a serious problem is detected. Screening tests an entire population. Testing refers to looking for a problem in individuals at a higher than usual risk; the words "screening" and "testing" are often used interchangeably, however.

Certain fetal abnormalities are most readily detected by measuring the amount of alpha-fetoprotein (AFP) in the mother's blood. Alpha-fetoprotein is a substance produced by the developing fetus in increasing amounts up to the fifteenth week of pregnancy. The level reaches a peak in the mother's blood between the twenty-eighth and thirty-second week of pregnancy. Abnormally high levels suggest that something may be wrong with the spinal cord or brain of the fetus. Abnormally low levels raise the suspicion that the fetus may have Down syndrome. To find out why an AFP test is abnormal, or for a variety of other reasons, one can also visualize the fetus through a radiation-free method of imaging called ultrasonography. Other test methods include amniocentesis, chorionic villus sampling, and removing a sample of fetal blood, all of which can be used to determine what genetic material a fetus has inherited.

THE ALPHA-FETOPROTEIN TEST

The AFP test is performed chiefly to detect defects in the neural tube, the structure that becomes the brain and spinal cord of the fetus. Normally, these two elements develop from a flat plate that folds upward and closes to form a tube. The neural tube closure starts at both ends and meets in the center. The tube closes by about the fourth week of development. Sometimes, though, neural tube closure fails at the head end, and a defect occurs in which the fetus has virtually no functioning brain. This condition is referred to as anencephaly; children with this affliction are usually born dead or die shortly after birth. There is no way to save them. The other common neural tube defect is spina bifida, in which the spinal cord is abnormal and the bony spine does not close completely or else closes abnormally.

The extensiveness of the impairment that results from spina bifida depends on the location and severity of the fault. In some cases a meningomyelocele, a sac containing undeveloped spinal cord and nerves, protrudes from the back. The most severely affected children are paralyzed, cannot control bowels or bladder, are mentally retarded, and have an abnormal accumulation of fluid in the brain called hydrocephalus. In less severe cases the child has little or no mental retardation and can learn to walk with braces. In its mildest form spina bifida generates no symptoms at all.

One reason why AFP screening is so important is that in many cases assessment and intervention in the first few days of life can dramatically affect the long-term outlook for the child born with spina bifida. If parents know in advance what kinds of problems the child may have, they can arrange for delivery and care in a center with specialized facilities and personnel. Ideally, for example, one would close a meningomyelocele surgically within the first 48 hours of life to avoid infection. The child should also be monitored for hydrocephalus, which must be treated surgically. A multidisciplinary team armed with skills in pediatrics, neurosurgery, pediatric surgery, urology, orthopedics, infectious diseases, mental health, and other areas as needed can get the infant off to the best possible start and provide support for the family. More information on neural tube defects is given in Chapter 3.

The first step in this particular screening program is to test the mother's blood for AFP during the second trimester. If the level is normal, no further testing needs to be done; if it is elevated, the neural tube may not have closed normally. Because of an open neural tube defect, AFP leaks into the amniotic fluid and from there, with some delay, into the mother's blood. One elevated AFP test does not necessarily mean that the fetus has a birth defect, however. A number of factors can explain a seemingly high value. The most common is miscalculation of the date of conception. Since the amount of AFP a fetus produces increases as it gets older, underestimating or overestimating its age can lead to a false value. The presence of more than one fetus can also lead to a seemingly abnormal value; so can other defects or other causes of fetal distress. If the first test is abnormally high, it should be repeated. If the second test again is high, the woman is usually referred for an ultrasound examination as the next step in determining the cause of the abnormality.

It is important to understand that the AFP test is not a general test for birth defects, nor a very specific one for defects of the neural tube. There is no discrete cutoff point that separates a normal test value from an abnormal one. The test results form a continuum, and sometimes it is impossible to distinguish a value that is at the high end of the normal scale from one that is at the low end of the elevated scale. Consequently, the AFP test will identify some normal fetuses as abnormal and will miss a defect in others. The confusion and distress caused by these difficulties in interpreting AFP test results are among the reasons some people object to routine use of the test. According to George Cunningham of the California Department of Health Services, the test still manages to pick up about 80 percent of neural tube defects and 20 percent of cases of Down syndrome.

Doctors usually describe the test results to their patients as a percentage of the average value for comparable women of the same race and body weight who take the test. According to Cunningham, an AFP value two and a half times normal is associated with a 14 percent chance of having a child with a neural tube defect. A value ten times normal is associated with an 88 percent chance of having a fetus with a neural tube defect or other serious abnormality. Sometimes a value this high can mean that the fetus is already dead. By itself, the test is less useful in detecting Down syndrome because the value that is abnormally low is not a great deal lower than normal.

Many present-day physicians routinely offer this simple, safe screening tool to all their pregnant patients. It is possible (but by no means certain) that if Amy had undergone AFP screening, she would have discovered before Ethan's birth that he had Down syndrome. The State of California has required since April 1986 that doctors offer their patients the option of participating in the state's AFP screening program. Cunningham reports in a July 1988 personal communication that more and more women are choosing to participate. The rate has increased from about 2,700 women per week when the program began to about 5,000 per week two years later. By May 1988 doctors in California had screened 447,000 pregnancies, about 60 percent of all pregnancies statewide.

A detailed analysis of the first year's 176,000 AFP screenings shows that 4.6 percent were positive. Further testing ultimately picked up 205 birth defects: 108 neural tube defects, 50 defects of the abdominal wall which cause the abdominal contents to be exposed, 17 cases of Down syndrome, and 30 cases of other chromosomal abnormalities. Overall this represents 11.6 abnormalities per 10,000 pregnancies screened. Ninety-one percent of the women bearing a fetus with a neural tube defect chose abortion, as did 40 percent of those with an abdominal wall defect, 78 percent of those with Down syndrome, and 63 percent of those with other chromosomal defects.

ULTRASONOGRAPHY

Ultrasonography, or ultrasound imaging, makes use of high-frequency sound waves to allow a skilled examiner to visualize the fetus while it is still in the mother's womb. Pulsed sound waves are beamed painlessly into the uterus through a transducer placed on the mother's abdomen. Tissues of various densities reflect the waves differently. The reflected waves are then visualized on a computer screen and printed out as a picture.

An ultrasound examination will often solve the mystery of an abnormal AFP test. If the woman is carrying more than one fetus, for example, this will be readily apparent. The ultrasound examination can also permit an accurate determination of the age of the fetus. Whereas obstetricians must rely on information the mothers give them and their physical examination to estimate age, the ultrasound permits precise measurements of fetal structures such as the diameter of the skull. Together with the clinical information these measurements enable the obstetrician to determine the age, which can then be correlated with the AFP values to achieve a more accurate picture of the status of the fetus.

Structural disorders (such as the size and location of spinal lesions) can be assessed via ultrasound, although accuracy depends on the age of the fetus, the technique used, and the experience and skill of the specialist. Anencephaly, for example, can be detected by the twelfth week, whereas spina bifida may not be visible even after the twentieth week, depending on the size and position of the fetus. Other disorders of the skeleton, central nervous system, kidneys, and urinary tract are often apparent on ultrasound.

If the elevated AFP test is not explained by ultrasonography, the doctor may recommend amniocentesis.

AMNIOCENTESIS

For more than twenty years doctors have been using amniocentesis to diagnose prenatal conditions. Both the amniotic fluid itself and the fetal cells it contains can provide useful information. To perform an amniocentesis, the physician inserts a needle through the mother's abdominal wall to withdraw a sample of amniotic fluid (Figure 3). A local anesthetic is applied first, to prevent discomfort to the mother. For maximum safety amniocentesis should be performed in conjunction with ultrasonography. The ultrasonographer can then locate the fetus and choose the best site for needle insertion, being careful to avoid puncturing the placenta, which can cause bleeding. Using what is called real-time ultrasound throughout the procedure, the doctor can keep the needle in view so that it does not harm the fetus.

Amniocentesis is performed at different times during the pregnancy, depending on the condition being assessed. We have already discussed karyotyping for chromosomal disorders. To rule out the presence of a neural tube defect, amniocentesis is performed between the sixteenth and twentieth weeks of pregnancy. The goal at this time is to measure the amounts of two substances in the amniotic fluid: alpha-fetoprotein and

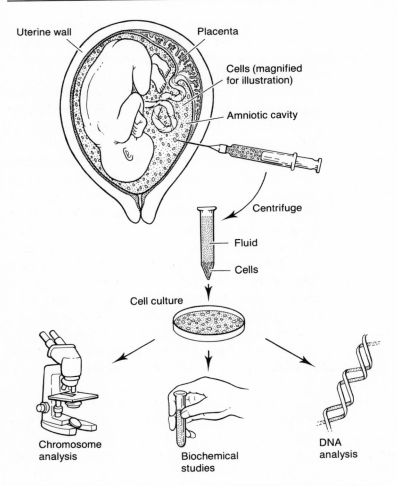

Figure 3. Amniocentesis is the most widely used technique for prenatal diagnosis in the second trimester of gestation. Guided by ultrasound, a needle is inserted through the mother's abdomen into the amniotic sac that surrounds the fetus. A small amount of amniotic fluid containing fetal cells is extracted and cultured. Cells and fluid are then analyzed for genetic abnormalities. Adapted from National Institute of General Medical Sciences, *The New Human Genetics,* NIH Publication 84-662, September 1984, p. 6.

acetylcholinesterase. Because the alpha-fetoprotein in amniotic fluid is released directly by the fetus, it is present in larger amounts and can be more accurately measured there than in the mother's blood serum.

Acetylcholinesterases, located primarily in the cells of the brain and central nervous system, are enzymes that break down the neurotransmitter acetylcholine. Developing and exposed nerve terminals release acetylcholinesterases, which pass into the amniotic fluid. Open neural tube defects, including anencephaly and spina bifida, are associated with elevated levels of acetylcholinesterases. If the amniotic fluid contains excessive levels of both AFP and acetylcholinesterases, the fetus almost certainly has a severe birth defect. If it does not, the fetus almost certainly does not have a severe birth defect of this sort.

Even though it is extremely helpful in diagnosing prenatal conditions, amniocentesis should not be undertaken lightly. Complications that affect either the mother or the fetus occur about 1 percent of the time. The intrusion of the needle into the sterile amniotic sac can cause infection, maternal bleeding, and injury to the fetus, and can even cause the fetus to be aborted. Most of the complications can be treated successfully, however.

An important drawback to amniocentesis is that it is rarely useful until the pregnancy is well established. When karyotyping is performed, it can take up to three weeks for technicians to grow enough cells in the laboratory to perform the test. Therefore, by the time the parents know if their child has a genetic disease, the pregnancy is well into the second trimester. Termination at this time requires inducing the delivery of a dead fetus. The parents have already felt it move, heard its heartbeat, and probably seen its image on ultrasound. Interrupting a pregnancy can cause long-lasting grief and depression. Furthermore, if laboratory error results in a sample that cannot be analyzed, by the time another sample is taken and the results are available, the fetus may be old enough to survive outside the womb in an advanced neonatal intensive care unit. Thus, the parents' options are severely curtailed.

Despite these disturbing considerations, terminating a pregnancy that involves a severely afflicted fetus or one with a fatal condition such as Tay-Sachs disease prevents a child's suffering, avoids prolonged distress to the family and others concerned with the child's care, and saves months or years of costly medical care. And the technology for interrupting pregnancies continues to improve, especially with regard to safety.

CHORIONIC VILLUS SAMPLING

Although doctors have less experience with this procedure than with amniocentesis, chorionic villus sampling offers hope of a first-trimester diagnosis of prenatal conditions. The chorion is a membrane that surrounds the fetus early in its gestation and later evolves into the placenta. Fingerlike projections (villi) of the chorion participate in blood transfer between mother and fetus. Cells from the chorionic villi contain the same genetic information as the fetus itself. One way to obtain samples of this tissue is for the doctor to insert a catheter through the vagina into the uterus. After using ultrasound to locate the fetus, the doctor applies suction to remove a sample of the villi (Figure 4). More and more obstetricians are obtaining the sample via a needle inserted into the abdomen, believing that this mode of entry is safer. Once the sample has been separated from the maternal cells, it can be analyzed as described below.

The excitement about chorionic villus sampling stems from the fact that it can be performed as early as nine weeks into pregnancy. In addition, a sample contains enough cells so that usually testing can be performed immediately, without taking time to grow more cells in the laboratory. Thus, parents can know as early as the tenth week of pregnancy whether the fetus

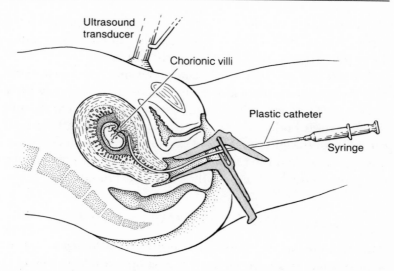

Figure 4. Chorionic villus sampling allows the detection of many genetic defects in the fetus as early as the ninth week of pregnancy. Fetal cells are suctioned out (through a thin tube threaded from the vagina and cervix into the uterus) from the chorionic villi, which are protrusions of a membrane (the chorion) that surrounds the developing fetus. The chorionic villi can also be reached by a needle inserted into the abdomen, as for amniocentesis. The harvested cells undergo chromosomal, DNA, and biochemical analysis, in much the same way as cells obtained by amniocentesis. Adapted from National Institute of General Medical Sciences, *The New Human Genetics,* NIH Publication 84-662, September 1984, p. 7.

has a genetic disease. If they opt to terminate the pregnancy, doing so in the first trimester lessens the physical and emotional trauma of the process.

Studies from China, Italy, and the United States indicate that the potential danger to the mother from chorionic villus sampling is minimal. The procedure carries about the same risk of miscarriage as amniocentesis.

PERCUTANEOUS UMBILICAL BLOOD SAMPLING

Until recently the only way to diagnose some conditions prenatally was by sampling blood from the fetus in a process called fetoscopy. Doctors generally prefer to avoid fetoscopy if at all possible because it can injure the fetus. A new method for sampling fetal blood—percutaneous umbilical blood sampling—has been developed in France. Doctors insert a needle through the abdomen and the uterus into the blood vessels of the umbilical cord. In this country Stuart Weiner of the University of Pennsylvania Medical School has had the most experience with the method, having used it on more than 200 fetuses since October 1985.

Not only can the availability of this blood facilitate the study of genetic conditions, it has also opened the door to treating conditions that affect either the expectant mother or the child. For example, in some cases doctors are able to give the fetus transfusions when its red blood cells are being destroyed by the mother's antibodies, a condition that arises when mother and child have different blood proteins (Rh factors). Usually such babies are treated after birth. The new method is not yet widely used, however, partly because of limited experience with it and partly because of the risk that infection will develop.

RECOMBINANT DNA ANALYSIS

Armed with the samples obtained from amniocentesis or chorionic villus sampling, doctors can go about determining the genetic well-being of the fetus. Although a comparatively small number of genetic diseases can be diagnosed by standard biochemical tests or chromosomal analysis, an increasing number rely on highly sophisticated, rapidly evolving technologies based on combining DNA from two different sources (recombinant DNA methods). Recombinant DNA is made by means of restriction enzymes, which cut DNA into pieces at specific locations because they recognize the nucleotide sequence there. These locations are called recognition sites. It is the nucleotide sequence that determines the amino acid sequence of the resulting protein. When a restriction enzyme cleaves a molecule, it leaves discrete ends on the DNA, which can then be joined to the ends of another piece of DNA.

In recent years scientists have learned how to splice and rejoin molecules, thus enabling them to diagnose more than 200 genetic diseases in the womb. In some cases they can determine directly if a fetus carries a gene for the disease; in other cases the diagnosis is made indirectly.

Direct Gene Detection

Suppose we wish to determine if a fetus carries a gene for a specific disorder in which the faulty gene results from the substitution of one nucleotide for another. One way is to use a gene probe. This is a short piece of single-strand DNA that is complementary to the DNA sequence being sought. Such a single strand will automatically search for and pair up with complementary strands.

To test fetal DNA, scientists first manufacture in the laboratory sequences of nucleotides that match the nucleotide sequences of both the normal and the flawed version of the gene in question. These probes are labeled radioactively for later identification on x-ray film. Next, the probes are added, one at a time, to a sample of fetal DNA. If the probe corresponding to the abnormal gene sticks to the fetal DNA, the fetus has inherited an abnormal gene; if the probe does not stick, the fetus has no abnormal gene for that condition. Similarly, if the probe corresponding to the normal gene sticks to the fetal DNA, the fetus has at least one normal gene for that trait.

Putting together information about whether the disease is transmitted in a dominant or a recessive fashion and the information gained from the use of probes, the doctors can then say whether the fetus has inherited the condition, is a carrier for that condition, or is free of it.

Gene probes can be used to diagnose phenylketonuria; hemophilia A; sickle cell disease; alpha-1-antitrypsin deficiency, an autosomally inherited disorder that causes severe lung disease in adults and liver disease in children; and thalassemia, a blood disorder characterized by anemia.

Another method of diagnosing genetic disorders directly is the Southern blot technique. The underlying principle here is that DNA fragments produced by restriction enzymes vary in length according to whether the fetal DNA sample contains the normal gene or the faulty gene. To determine these variations, scientists use gene probes. They cut up the DNA with restriction enzymes, treat the resulting pieces so that they are single stranded rather than double stranded, then separate the fragments by size using a process called electrophoresis. With radioactively labeled probes and specially treated filter paper, they can identify the normal or abnormal genes from the length of the lines produced.

Hemoglobin disorders lend themselves particularly well to detection by Southern blot analysis. Thalassemia, for example, is caused by the absence of part of the gene sequence. The fragment that shows up on the blot is smaller than normal or may not appear at all. Sickle cell disease is also easy to detect, because the DNA error that causes it occurs in the middle of the site of the usual cut by a restriction enzyme. Because the restriction enzyme does not break the DNA normally in a case of sickle cell disease the result will be one long fragment of 1,350 base pairs, rather than two shorter ones. A carrier of sickle cell disease would be identified by this test as well, since the appearance of a long band as well as the two shorter ones would indicate the presence of one normal gene and one defective gene.

The Indirect Method

Direct gene detection is the ideal, and most accurate, form of recombinant DNA technology for diagnosing genetic disorders prenatally. Unfortunately, in only a small number of diseases is the exact location and composition of the faulty gene known at this time. For other conditions one must resort to an indirect diagnostic method based on restriction fragment-length polymorphisms, or RFLPs. Although this multisyllabic phrase may suggest a very complicated notion, the concept behind it is quite simple. It reflects the fact that the pieces of DNA produced by restriction enzymes vary in length naturally among different members of a family.

Scientists have learned that if an RFLP is close to a disease-producing gene on a chromosome, a person is very likely to inherit both the RFLP and the gene. By analyzing the DNA segments produced by both healthy members of a family and those affected by the genetic disease in question, they can determine which is the "healthy pattern" and which is the "affected pattern." If they then compare the segments produced by the DNA of a fetus, they can say with reasonable certainty whether or not the fetus carries the gene for the disease. The accuracy of the test depends on how closely linked the RFLP and the gene are.

The first disease to be diagnosed in this way was Huntington's, the dread degenerative disease of the central nervous system. There is much that scientists do not yet know about Huntington's disease. They do not fully understand the biochemical dysfunctions that underlie it. Nor do they understand what goes wrong in the body to cause it. Thanks to the persistent work of Nancy Wexler and James Gusella, however, most people who carry the gene can now be identified.

Gusella, who published a report of his work in 1983, first used restriction enzymes to digest the DNA of patients with Huntington's disease. He then separated the resulting fragments by length and used radioactive probes to detect the suspected region of DNA. He found that DNA from different people produced fragments of different sizes because of insertions or deletions of nucleotides in the DNA in the recognition sites of restriction enzymes.

Wexler and Gusella took their study to Lake Maracaibo in Venezuela, where more than a thousand interrelated people are at risk for developing Huntington's disease. Over a period of several years they found that members of the extended family who developed the condition produced specific RFLPs, whereas those who did not have the disease produced different fragments. Although they have yet to find the precise location of the gene, they have narrowed it down to a small area on chromosome 4 and can now diagnose with 95 percent certainty whether a person or a fetus has the gene.

The RFLP-based test for Huntington's disease is currently available at a small number of centers in the United States. Theoretically, people at risk because they have an affected parent can go there and find out whether or not they too have the gene for this autosomal-dominant inherited condition. The test can also be used for prenatal diagnosis—but a fetus can only have the gene if one of its parents does too. Many people opt not to obtain this information. They prefer to live with uncertainty rather than ascertain that they will develop this tragic disease for which there is no cure. Among those who choose to make the determination, 50 percent will be reassured that they do not carry the gene, and their lives will be changed for the better. For the other 50 percent, the impact of learning that they carry the gene is problematic.

Familial hypercholesterolemia and sickle cell disease can also be diagnosed by means of RFLPs. Although family studies are necessary to diagnose familial hypercholesterolemia so that the normal and abnormal fragment lengths can be determined, diagnosing sickle cell disease does not require this information, for the genetic flaw occurs in the restriction enzyme's recognition site. Therefore, the restriction enzyme does not cleave the DNA at this location of people with this condition, whereas it *will* cleave the DNA of normal people. The difference between one fragment and two fragments can be quickly determined in the laboratory, in many centers permitting a diagnosis the same day a sample is received.

CARRIER SCREENING

Carrier screening is the process of identifying, before a pregnancy takes place, whether one or both members of a couple carry a gene for an autosomal-recessive or X-linked disorder. By means of biochemical analyses for enzymes or hemoglobin types, or the recombinant DNA techniques described above, carrier screening is useful in conditions such as Tay-Sachs disease, sickle cell disease, some forms of thalassemia, and Duchenne's muscular dystrophy, although the tests for the last disease are not accurate in all cases. In light of the recent identification of the gene for cystic fibrosis, some carriers with no family history of the disease can now be identified as well. Tests for the general population remain to be developed. The information from carrier screening is particularly useful in preventing the birth of the first affected child to a couple who, without screening, would be unaware of their risk.

CHAPTER 3

Five Common Genetic Diseases

Today some 250 genetic diseases and birth defects can be diagnosed prenatally. Although the vast majority of prenatal tests serve to reassure parents that their unborn baby is free of the suspected condition, sometimes the tests identify a baby who is seriously ill. At this point the parents' choice is between preparing for the birth of an afflicted child and ending the pregnancy. Only personal experience can give a realistic appraisal of what life with a serious genetic disease means; still, to assist in one of the most formidable of life's choices we attempt in this chapter to describe the genetics, characteristics, and outlook for individuals with the five most common genetic diseases. The appendix will aid the reader in locating similar information on some of the other genetic diseases and defects.

DOWN SYNDROME

Down syndrome is the most common chromosomal disorder. If nothing is done to prevent the birth of children with this condition, it affects about 1 in 1,000 babies born each year in the United States, for an annual total of about 3,500 babies. The incidence rises with the mother's age, rising from 1 in 2,000 for women in their early twenties to about 1 in 350 for women of thirty-five. By the time a woman reaches forty, the chances are about 1 in 100 that her pregnancy will be affected by this abnormality of the gene-containing bodies, the chromosomes.

Because they possess an extra twenty-first chromosome, children with this condition share certain characteristics; foremost among them is mental retardation. Brain development and maturation are progressive processes: as they occur, a child can perform increasingly complex tasks. From smiling, sitting up, and walking, he or she moves to talking, caring for personal needs, reading, and problem solving. For the child with Down syndrome, brain development is slow and abnormal. The afflicted youngster is capable of the full range of emotions and can love and feel joy and pride in accomplishment. Although affection, attention, and stimulation help the child a great deal, normal mental functioning is not attainable.

Particularly in their early years, children with Down syndrome may not seem much different from other children. They can often learn to feed and dress themselves and perform simple repetitive jobs like setting the table. Their peak intellectual capacity, however, is most often that of a six- or seven-year-old child. Personally and socially, they function at a slightly higher level. Although we must be cautious about stereotypes, individuals with Down syndrome tend to enjoy being with people, seem happy much of the time, and fit in with social units such as their family, day-care center, and school group.

The lives of children and young adults with Down syndrome seem to be simpler than normal. Their emotions, including their sexual feelings, appear less intense. Parents often find that their children have a definite preference about their activities and can be quite stubborn. Many enjoy music and playing in the water. Talking, a complex task intellectually, comes later for children with Down syndrome than for others. Many do not say their first words until they are two or three years old.

The degree of mental retardation of people with Down syndrome ranges from severe to moderate. So, too, their physical traits and disabilities run along a spectrum from severe or very noticeable to not present at all. About a third of the children born with this affliction die shortly after birth or in early childhood, usually because of severe heart defects. Typical of the life-threatening defects of the heart is the presence of an opening between the two sides, which can impede the heart's ability to pump oxygen-rich blood to vital organs and leave the baby short of energy. Repairing these defects requires major surgery; a frail child may not be able to withstand the trauma. Another potential problem for children with Down syndrome is that they are more vulnerable to respiratory and other infections than normal children. But unless they also have severe heart problems or other major defects, the family physician or pediatrician can usually manage the children's everyday medical needs.

Because of their extra chromosome, children with Down syndrome have certain physical traits that make them easily recognizable. Their eyes tend to slant upward, and they may have small skin folds at the inside corners of their eyes. The resulting Asian-like appearance accounts for the term "mongolism," which was formerly used to designate the disease.

As Ethan's physician noticed when he was born, children with Down syndrome tend to have poor muscle tone; doctors refer to them as being "floppy," a condition that usually improves as the child gets older. The back of the head is flatter than usual, and the head in general is smaller than normal. The child's nose has a low bridge; the tongue tends to protrude somewhat because it is larger than usual. The hands usually are shorter and broader than normal and have a single crease across the upper palm instead of two. Finally, children with Down syndrome tend to be short and stocky.

As they become teenagers, they tend to develop sexually later than usual and incompletely. Boys, for example, tend to have less facial hair; girls' breasts may not develop fully. Men with Down syndrome appear to be sterile, but some women have had children. The child of a person with Down syndrome has a fifty-fifty chance of also having Down syndrome, since he or she has a fifty-fifty chance of inheriting two joined twenty-first chromosomes from the mother and one from the father. Because of their naivete and trusting nature, people with Down syndrome need protection from sexual exploitation.

At birth, babies with Down syndrome are less mature than normal infants but physically they age more rapidly than normal, and after they reach forty, their mortality increases sharply. Pneumonia is often the cause of death.

A major concern of the parents of children with Down syndrome is how to provide a secure future for them. Children raised at home in their early years tend to progress more quickly than those raised in institutions. But by the time the children reach preschool age, they often have difficulty finding playmates. To all intents and purposes, the person with Down syndrome will never achieve a completely independent lifestyle and will always need supervision.

Families find different ways of working out these problems. A number of day-care centers and special preschool programs are designed for children with Down syndrome. For families that do not have the emotional or financial resources to care for their young children at home, foster homes, group homes, and institutions are available. Infant stimulation programs, support groups, special-education facilities, recreational programs, day programs, and residential settings are options to consider. Many communities have developed resources that were not available just a few years ago.

SICKLE CELL DISEASE

As we have seen, sickle cell disease is a disorder of red blood cells caused by the presence of an abnormal amino acid in one of the chains of the hemoglobin molecule. Hemoglobin is the pigment that gives red blood cells their color; the job of the red blood cells is to carry oxygen. As a result of the abnormal hemoglobin, the affected person's red blood cells, instead of being round, sometimes (especially if oxygen in the blood is low) become sickle or crescent shaped, as observed under the microscope (Figure 5). Cells of this shape tend to become trapped and destroyed in the spleen. With too few red blood cells the affected person becomes anemic, is often short of breath, and tires easily.

Sickle cells may also clog small blood vessels, causing tissues fed by these vessels to wither. People with sickle cell disease are more likely than normal people to develop infections, and their physical growth and development may be slowed. Infections can further deplete the red blood cell supply, intensifying the anemia. When the anemia becomes severe, the white part of the eye may become yellow from the presence of yellow chemicals formed by the destruction of hemoglobin, which then circulate in the blood. Other troublesome aspects of this condition include a high risk of stroke, damage to the retina, and skin ulcers.

Although most people with sickle cell disease can function

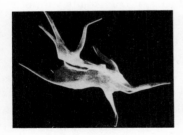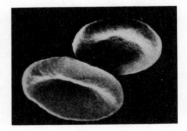

Figure 5. An autosomal-recessive disorder, sickle cell disease is caused by the mutation of a single nucleotide in the beta-globin gene. The abnormal beta-globin chains cause the red blood cells to become crescent or sickle shaped (at left); two normal cells are shown at right for comparison. Photos by Marcel Bessis.

normally much of the time, the disease sometimes proves disabling or fatal for children and young adults. The specific symptoms and their degree vary from person to person. Extremely painful episodes called sickle cell crises are likely to punctuate the course of the illness. When these occur, the sickled cells become stuck in the blood vessels; other cells pile up behind them until the vessels become completely blocked. These logjams occur in bones and other organs of the abdomen and chest, depriving the tissues of oxygen. Such episodes can permanently damage the brain, lungs, and kidneys. A child may feel fine some of the time, yet be absent from school for considerable periods because of the need for hospitalization. Adults frequently are unable to hold full-time jobs.

To develop this disease, which is inherited in an autosomal-recessive fashion, a child must inherit a sickle cell gene from each parent. The March of Dimes Birth Defects Foundation estimates that 1 in 10 African-Americans carries the gene, or "has the sickle cell trait." People with the trait rarely show symptoms of anemia unless they are subjected to high altitudes or other environments very low in oxygen.

According to the March of Dimes, about 1 in 400 to 600 African-Americans and 1 in 1,000 to 1,500 Hispanics inherit two genes for sickle cell hemoglobin and therefore develop the disease. A small percentage of people of Arabic, Greek, Maltese, Sicilian, Sardinian, Turkish, and southern Asian ancestry are also affected. The sickle cell gene in a single dose is believed to confer on those who have it an increased resistance to certain forms of malaria, explaining the prevalence of sickle cell disease in areas of the world that previously had or still have a great deal of malaria.

Prospective parents who are at risk of passing on the sickle cell gene, either because of their ancestry or because they have a relative with sickle cell disease, should before they have children consider determining if they carry the trait; a simple blood test identifies carriers. If both parents carry the gene and pregnancy occurs, they may want to consider prenatal testing. Sickle cell disease can be diagnosed by chorionic villus sampling in the first trimester of a pregnancy, and by amniocentesis at about the sixteenth week via direct gene analysis. Community programs for carrier screening are now common.

Some children inherit one sickle cell gene plus a gene for another disease that affects the red blood cells, such as thalassemia. These combinations can cause anemia and sickling, but in general are less troublesome than sickle cell disease. Carriers of genes for these conditions can be detected by restriction fragment-length polymorphism studies.

At this time doctors do not know how to prevent the sickling of red blood cells. Research is in process to find a way, as well as to learn how to remove excess iron from the bodies of people with sickle cell disease, who must receive frequent transfusions. The iron, which comes from the breakdown of red blood cells, can gradually build up and interfere with the functioning of vital organs. Screening of newborn babies is recommended, because early medical treatment can reduce suffering and improve the outcome for babies with sickle cell disease.

NEURAL TUBE DEFECTS

Defects of the neural tube are the most common serious birth defects in the United States, affecting 1 to 2 children in 1,000 live births. Anencephaly, a defect in which the child has no functioning brain, is fatal within days. But most children with spina bifida survive.

Spina bifida is thought to result from a combination of genetic and environmental influences. A woman who has already given birth to a child with spina bifida has a 2.5 to 5 percent risk of having a second child with the problem. The incidence of spina bifida is higher in certain geographic and ethnic groups, such as people from Northern Ireland and Wales and Appalachians in the United States. And whites give birth to children with neural tube defects twice as often as African-Americans. The lack of certain nutrients is thought to contribute; in some studies poor women gave birth to children with neural tube defects more often than others, as did women who conceived in the winter and early spring when fresh fruits and vegetables are scarce. Deficiencies of folic acid, which is found in leafy green vegetables, appear to be a factor. Vitamin supplements before conception and during pregnancy may prove helpful in preventing spina bifida in those genetically predisposed to it, but research in this area is inconclusive.

In spina bifida the spinal cord forms abnormally, with the tissue that covers the cord or the cord itself displaced outside the spinal canal. A mild form is called spina bifida occulta: the defect is covered by skin and the affected person may have few or no symptoms at all. The visible forms are referred to as spina bifida manifesta. The most common type is characterized by a meningomyelocele that protrudes from the back. A less common form is a meningocele, in which a sac containing the membranes that usually envelop the brain and spinal cord protrudes through a defect in the skull or vertebral column.

The location of the spinal defect determines the type and extent of disability, since all the nerves below the sac are usually damaged. The spinal column contains 31 groups of nerves. At the top are the cervical nerves, which carry messages to the upper part of the body, including the arms and hands. Then come the thoracic nerves, which transmit signals from the breastbone to the abdomen and part of the arms. Next come the lumbar nerves, which serve the hips, front of the legs, and top of the feet. Lower down are the sacral nerves, which supply the lower legs, feet, back of the legs, bladder, rectum, and genitals. Finally, the coccygeal nerve supplies the skin and supporting muscles around the anus.

Although babies with spina bifida are often hydrocephalic, about 70 percent of children with spina bifida have normal intelligence and can go to conventional schools when they are old enough. Early medical attention is *imperative*. To avoid infection, the doctor must close any open lesion of the spinal cord within the first two days of life. If the baby shows physical signs of hydrocephalus, or if ultrasound examination or x-rays indicate that it is present, a tube must be implanted in a cavity in the brain during the first few days to drain the excess fluid into the abdomen or heart in an effort to prevent damage to the brain from the pressure of the fluid. These shunts must be replaced as the child grows.

Children with spina bifida will come to know an awesome number of medical specialists. In the first hours of life they will meet neurosurgeons, who specialize in the care of damaged brain and spinal tissue. They will come to know urologists and gastroenterologists, who treat kidney and bowel problems, respectively. Later they will visit orthopedists, who deal with the spine, muscles, bones, and joints. Physical therapists and nurses will improve their mobility with exercises and coordinate their care. Mental health professionals can help them make the most of their lives and reach their potential, as well as providing the family with information about community resources.

People with many varieties of neural tube defects often have incompletely developed or damaged nerves supplying the legs, bladder, and bowel. The manifestations are muscle paralysis, lack of bladder and bowel control, loss of skin sensation, and spinal and limb deformities.

Bladder and bowel control are perhaps the most difficult aspects of spina bifida for the affected person. Because the relevant nerves are damaged, children have no way of knowing when their bladders are full, they cannot release their urine completely, or they cannot stop the flow. As a result, urine can accumulate in the bladder and back up into the kidneys, which are then prone to infection. The standard method of managing this problem and preventing damage to the urinary system is clean, intermittent catheterization. A tube is inserted into the urethra to drain urine from the bladder every three to four hours. Children can often learn to do this themselves, and schools are now required to provide this service for those who cannot.

Lack of bowel control, because of its social implications, is also a problem for people with spina bifida. Dietary management, establishing specific times for moving the bowels, and medication are the basic remedies suggested, but even adults may require diapers.

The ability of the person with spina bifida to get around depends by and large on the location and extent of damage and the person's body build. Some people are able to get around with braces; others are restricted to wheelchairs. A mix of surgery, splinting, braces, and exercises to stretch and strengthen muscles may also assist in maximizing this ability.

Women with spina bifida frequently are able to bear children, but their offspring face a 4 to 5 percent chance of having the same genetic defect. Prenatal screening, starting with the alpha-fetoprotein test, is quite effective in identifying this condition. About 60 percent of the men with spina bifida have no sexual impairment and can father children.

CYSTIC FIBROSIS

Cystic fibrosis (CF) is the most common disease of Caucasians that is caused by a single gene present in double dose. About 15 million Americans, or 5 percent of the U.S. population, carry the gene. About 30,000 have CF, and among Caucasians it occurs roughly once in 1,600 births. It is inherited in an autosomal-recessive way, which means that to develop CF a child must receive a gene for it from each parent.

Until very recently, prenatal diagnosis of cystic fibrosis was possible only for families who already had a member with the disease. The diagnosis was based on restriction fragment-length polymorphism studies, described in Chapter 2. Then, in September 1989, researchers from centers in Canada and the United States announced that they had found the long-sought gene for cystic fibrosis.[1]

Using a technique called chromosome walking and jumping, they had systematically traversed chromosome 7, jumping over unhelpful areas of DNA, until they found the gene on the chromosome's long arm. Once the gene had been located, attention focused on determining what was wrong with it. The investigators learned that the predominant mutation, or genetic abnormality, that causes cystic fibrosis results from a deletion of three nucleotides that code for the amino acid phenylalanine. Because this amino acid does not get added to the protein chain, the faulty protein impairs salt and chloride transportation, which partially explains why individuals with cystic fibrosis have excessively salty sweat.

Although identification of the gene that causes cystic fibrosis is a major advance, this mutation occurs in only about 68 percent of people with cystic fibrosis. Therefore, direct gene testing of the population at large would miss many carriers. For prenatal diagnosis in families with a history of the disease, however, direct testing for cystic fibrosis is already under way—supplemented when necessary by restriction fragment-length polymorphism studies. This combined approach provides an answer within 24 hours for many families.

Peter Ray, who heads the prenatal diagnosis laboratory at the

1. Johanna M. Rommens, Michael C. Iannuzzi, Bat-Sheva Kerem et al., "Identification of the Cystic Fibrosis Gene: Chromosome Walking and Jumping," *Science* 245 (1989): 1059–65; John R. Riordan, Johanna M. Rommens, Bat-Sheva Kerem et al., "Identification of the Cystic Fibrosis Gene: Cloning and Characterization of Complementary DNA," *Science* 245 (1989): 1066–73; and Bat-Sheva Kerem, Johanna M. Rommens, Janet A. Buchanan et al., "Identification of the Cystic Fibrosis Gene: Genetic Analysis," *Science* 245 (1989): 1073–80.

Hospital for Sick Children in Toronto, where much of this path-breaking research took place, anticipates that the remaining mutations will be found within the year, long before funding and facilities become available to provide mass screening. Identification of the mutations that cause cystic fibrosis will also lead to better understanding of the disease and development of more effective treatments than are presently available.

Forty years ago most children with CF died in early childhood. Now, thanks to medical advances, more than half live into their twenties and 40 percent live to the age of thirty.

The predominant medical problems of people with CF are progressive lung obstruction and digestive problems caused by the body's inability to absorb fat and protein. The researchers who found the cystic fibrosis gene believe that patients with digestive problems in addition to their lung disease have somewhat different flaws in their genes than those without digestive problems. A baby born with CF may seem perfectly normal at first. The symptoms of CF, which may not appear until later in childhood, are similar to those of many other pulmonary and digestive conditions: persistent cough, wheezing, pneumonia, poor weight gain, and bulky, foul-smelling stools. Because of the ambiguity of these symptoms, a diagnosis may not be made for a number of years. By that time other children with the disease may have been born into the family.

The progressive lung obstruction of CF is caused by excessive secretion of thick, choking mucus that blocks airways and predisposes to respiratory infections. This problem is complicated by the fact that people with CF cannot fight off infections the way normal people can. The respiratory infections that used to kill most children with CF now can usually be controlled with antibiotics, however. Children may need to go into the hospital periodically for two to three weeks to receive intravenous antibiotics. Some children and young adults stay on oral antibiotics indefinitely.

Regular physical therapy for the chest is critical to loosen mucus so that the person with CF can cough it up and minimize the likelihood of respiratory infection. The therapy is commonly carried out in the form of bronchial, or postural, drainage, which aims to help the mucus flow from the small airways into the large airways. The individual lies or sits in various positions while the area is slapped to stimulate the movement of secretions. Children need the help of an adult, but adults can often perform much of the therapy themselves.

Excessive mucus also impedes the digestive process because it blocks the ducts or openings of the pancreas, an organ that provides the enzymes needed to digest food. To relieve the pain, gas, and diarrhea that result from the inability of the pancreatic enzymes to do their job, people with CF take pancreatic enzyme replacement therapy—sometimes as many as thirty or forty capsules a day, with meals and snacks. The number of capsules needed varies with the person's condition and the content of the meal.

Until recently people with CF were told to avoid fatty food and restrict their diet. Most doctors no longer make this recommendation because patients need the fat to increase their weight and strength. In fact, people with CF require more than the daily allowance of calories recommended for normal people since they must work so hard to breathe. Not taking in enough nutrients makes them less able to fight off infection and weakens their already debilitated respiratory muscles. To ensure adequate nutrition, some people with CF require that a high-calorie formula be infused by a tube through the stomach or a nasogastric tube passing from the nose to the stomach via the esophagus.

As they enter their teens, adolescents with CF may be late in developing secondary sexual traits and may be smaller than their peers. In particular, girls often do not have enough body fat to permit menstruation at the usual age. Teens may find breathing difficult and they may feel constantly tired. High school students must plan for the future under the cloud of not knowing if they will live to be thirty and knowing that in all likelihood they will not live beyond their forties.

As they enter young adulthood, these teenagers tend to develop complications, including extensive polyps in the nose and curvature of the spine. As the disease inexorably progresses, they must cope with increasing dependence on others. Women may be capable of bearing children, but they often emerge from pregnancy with diminished lung function. Although they pass on one CF gene to each child, their children will be normal unless the father is a CF carrier. Males with CF tend to be sterile.

There is no cure for cystic fibrosis. Treatment is aimed at easing symptoms and preventing complications. At times the regimen is overwhelming, to the point that life may seem to revolve around the illness. The families of those with CF need many support services from the community.

TAY-SACHS DISEASE

The lives of children born with Tay-Sachs disease are short and tragic and cause heartbreak for parents who can do nothing to stop their children's progressive, terminal deterioration. Infants with this condition usually seem fine at birth. By the age of about six months parents notice that the children's muscles seem to weaken and the babies lose the ability to hold up their head or sit up. At about that time an ophthalmologist can usually find a characteristic red spot on the retina in the back of the eye. As the disease progresses, the children regress mentally and physically. Toward the end they become severely retarded, lose their vision, cannot control their movements, and develop seizures. Death usually comes by about four years of age.

As we have seen, Tay-Sachs disease is caused by a deficiency of hexosaminidase A, an enzyme whose job it is to break down complex molecules derived from the central nervous system. Because of the enzyme deficiency, the molecules do not break down and instead accumulate in the cells, causing progressive neurological disease (see Figure 6). Tay-Sachs occurs most commonly among Ashkenazi Jews of Eastern European ancestry. Like cystic fibrosis and sickle cell disease, it is inherited in an autosomal-recessive fashion. A simple, inexpensive blood test can detect carriers, and amniocentesis can be used to diagnose Tay-Sachs disease prenatally, because the cells from normal fetuses produce the enzyme hexosaminidase A and the cells from affected fetuses do not.

Because Tay-Sachs disease occurs in such a discrete population, carrier screening has been extremely successful in reducing the number of babies born with it. Eve Nichols notes in *Human Gene Therapy* that in the late 1980s fewer than 10 babies with Tay-Sachs disease were born each year in the United States, compared with 50 to 100 in 1970. Screening programs among Ashkenazi Jews have identified more than 15,000 carriers (1 of every 25 persons tested) and more than 800 couples at risk of bearing a Tay-Sachs child.

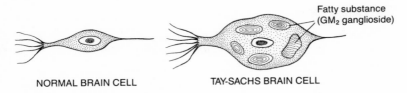

Fatty substance
(GM$_2$ ganglioside)

NORMAL BRAIN CELL   TAY-SACHS BRAIN CELL

Figure 6. A fatal genetic disorder in children, Tay-Sachs disease causes progressive destruction of the central nervous system. Children with the disease lack the enzyme hexosaminidase A. Without it, a fatty substance called GM$_2$ ganglioside accumulates and destroys the nerve cells in the brain.

One group of traditional Jews in New York City has found a particularly creative screening method.[2] In this Orthodox culture marriages are still arranged by a matchmaker, and the community finds contraception and abortion unacceptable. Yet one rabbi, who had lost four children to Tay-Sachs disease, knew that the only way to avert this devastating condition was to prevent marriages between carriers. Since the community believed that taking the carrier test would stigmatize families, the members were opting not to participate. The rabbi's solution was to arrange for people to identify themselves only by number when they went to the screening center. Later the matchmaker was told the test results for a prospective couple. If neither or only one was a carrier, the marriage could proceed. If both were carriers, and therefore at risk for bearing children with Tay-Sachs disease, she told the families to contact the screening center. Consequently, it was only if they were matched with another carrier that individuals would learn that they themselves were carriers. They could then look for a new spouse without the community at large knowing the reason.

The program, known as Chevra Dor Yeshorim (Association of the Upright Generation), began in 1983. By 1987 more than 4,000 people had been tested and the marriage of six pairs of carriers had been avoided. All the carriers were subsequently paired with noncarriers. Not a single child has been born with Tay-Sachs disease in this community.

2. See Beverly Merz, "Matchmaking Scheme Solves Tay-Sachs Problem," *Journal of the American Medical Association* 258 (1987): 2636–39.

CHAPTER 4

Ethical Concerns

On May 12, 1988, *New York Times* columnist Anna Quindlen explained publicly why she would not be undergoing amniocentesis. Almost thirty-six and the mother of two young sons, she realized that she faced a substantial risk of giving birth to a child with Down syndrome. Yet she decided not to have amniocentesis because she would not submit to an abortion even if the tests showed the child to have this chromosomal disorder. In a column entitled "The Child I Carry Is Wanted, Healthy or Not," she wrote: "Perhaps if this child were unwanted, I could think of it as a fetus. But my children—three of them now— have all been wanted; they were babies from the moment I knew they were coming." She asked herself what condition in her pregnancy would be a "sufficient impediment" to cause her to abort it. Down syndrome and spina bifida did not fall into that category, although she was uncertain about what she would do if she knew that the child had Tay-Sachs disease or schizophrenia or autism, the last two of which she described as her "two personal demons."

Urged by her doctor to consider that if she had an impaired child who needed her constant attention, she might have less time for her other children, she did think about this aspect. But she dismissed that as an argument for undergoing amniocentesis, reasoning that "having more than one child always means a willingness either to give less to the others or to stretch yourself more."

Quindlen's thoughtful column elicited a stream of letters, some of which were printed on the following June 9. Among them was one from a mother of three children, the eldest of whom has Down syndrome. In her two subsequent pregnancies, she wrote, she had undergone amniocentesis and would have chosen abortion had the tests indicated the presence of Down syndrome. She made this decision because of the quality of life facing her retarded child. Her daughter, she noted, "despite bountiful love and support within the family, must venture forth and face life as a label . . . I would have wished her a life with less pain, both physical—a result of several corrective surgeries—and the endless other. I would have wished her better answers to questions about why she won't go to college like her sisters, or drive a car, or whether she will have meaningful work or live on her own."

Another letter writer, the twin of a child with a small brain (a condition known as microencephaly), accused Quindlen of writing about "a situation that she has never experienced: the rearing of a hopelessly ill child." The writer elaborated: "In 28 years my mother never had a respite from travail. Her child was constantly ill, with no control over his bodily functions. For 28 years, my father worked as many as three jobs at once because his son was never approved for medical insurance."

Yet another response described Quindlen's action as selfish, in that she had taken it upon herself to decide how much her child, if born, would endure. The writer was thirty-eight and pregnant with her first child. She had undergone prenatal screening for Down syndrome and spina bifida and had been assured that her child did not have these conditions. She asked, "Does [Quindlen] really believe that not having tests after the age of thirty-five, when women automatically go into the high-risk pregnancy category, shows that she wants her baby more than I want mine?"

This emotional exchange highlights one of the most important considerations that must be taken into account if prenatal diagnostic technologies are to be used ethically: prenatal screening is a highly personal matter about which people, because of their varied religious beliefs and life experiences, harbor strong feelings and convictions. Ideally, the genetic counseling process is one in which the counselor provides truthful, understandable information to prospective parents about the potential and limitations of the available tests, so that they can make informed decisions in keeping with their values. The counselor then honors and supports their choices, and protects their privacy. Some people, like Anna Quindlen, will decide not to avail themselves of all possible tests. Others, like some of those who responded so fervently, will want every bit of information they can collect.

Ironically, in light of the intensely personal nature of the matter, a woman may find that many other parties become involved in her decision-making process, either directly or indirectly. As society struggles to incorporate the new technologies, which though evolving rapidly are scarce and expensive, she interacts with health care providers, who are entitled, just as she is, to act in accordance with their own moral code (but who have the obligation to grant a referral if provider and patient differ fundamentally). Furthermore, decisions made by the prospective parents and the health care providers affect the well-being of the fetus, who cannot voice its own values and preferences but who in turn affects the well-being of the family—and who, in some cases, becomes a public charge.

On a larger scale, health planners and legislators must weigh investment in the facilities and personnel required to prevent or control genetic diseases against the need to provide services for those who are born with these debilitating conditions. In addition, the new diagnostic technologies are used within a health care system that is influenced by biases in the society at large. Clearly identifiable groups within the society (minorities, for example) have less access to services and to prenatal care. These issues are especially relevant to prenatal diagnosis, inasmuch as some of the most common genetic diseases occur more frequently in certain ethnic groups (sickle cell disease in African-Americans, for instance).

GENDER SCREENING

Medical geneticists themselves are troubled by the use of prenatal diagnostic technologies to determine the sex of the fetus, so that a healthy fetus of the "wrong" (usually female) sex can be aborted. In a survey of attitudes among 677 medical geneticists in 18 nations completed in 1987, this issue was identified as the source of the greatest ethical conflict to the largest number of respondents in a questionnaire about the difficult choices that arise when treating patients. Overall, 42 percent of those surveyed said that they would either perform prenatal diagnosis for sex selection or refer the couple to another medical geneticist who would. In the United States, Hungary, and India, a majority would perform the test. The geneticists in the United States cited respect for parental autonomy as their predominant reason; in Hungary, all 15 who supported the practice did so to prevent the otherwise certain abortion of a normal fetus, because the parents preferred no child to one of the unwanted sex.

Dorothy Wertz and John Fletcher, who carried out the survey, commented that the respondents who would perform prenatal diagnosis for sex selection, or refer patients to someone who would, appeared to be unaware of the social consequences of using prenatal diagnosis for this purpose, in terms of either overloading the health care system or fostering sexist attitudes. Rather, they saw it as "an extension of families' self-evident right to determine the number, spacing, and quality of their children." [1]

In the United States the President's Commission for the Study of Ethical Problems in Medicine and Biomedical and Behavioral Research, on the other hand, described prenatal diagnosis for sexual selection as "an affront to the notion of human equality." It noted that "if it became an accepted practice, the selection of sons in preference to daughters would be yet another means of assigning a greater social value to one sex over the other and of perpetuating the historical discrimination against women."

The commission took issue with the whole notion of picking and choosing the characteristics one wants in one's children. "Taken to an extreme," it noted, "this attitude treats a child as an artifact and the reproductive process as a chance to design and produce human beings according to parental standards of excellence" rather than seeing prenatal screening as a tool to avoid disability or to improve the well-being of a fetus. [2]

The *New York Times* in 1988 reported that the western Indian state of Maharashtra, which includes Bombay, had recently banned the use of prenatal tests to determine a child's sex. Some hospitals and clinics had made no attempt to hide the economic advantages to a family of having boys rather than girls, for whom a dowry must be provided. The use of amni-

1. Dorothy C. Wertz and John C. Fletcher, "Attitudes of Genetic Counselors: A Multinational Survey," *American Journal of Human Genetics* 42 (1988): 592–600.

2. President's Commission for the Study of Ethical Problems in Medicine and Biomedical and Behavioral Research, *Screening and Counseling for Genetic Conditions: A Report on the Ethical, Social and Legal Implications of Genetic Screening, Counseling, and Education Programs* (Washington, D.C.: Government Printing Office, 1983), pp. 57, 58.

a sex-determination test had been advertised with
n as "Better to spend 500 rupees now than 50,000
r." To undergo amniocentesis in Maharashtra today,
must be at least thirty-five years old or have a medical or family history suggesting that her fetus may inherit a genetic disease or defect.[3] In the United States the President's Commission stopped short of urging a legal prohibition of this practice, noting that state involvement in such a personal matter might be more offensive than the practice itself.

SOCIAL AND ECONOMIC PROBLEMS

In fact, the programs to screen for sickle cell carriers mandated by some state governments in this country in the early 1970s are notable examples of the strong feelings that unwanted government intervention can engender and the harm that can be caused by misinformed and misguided legislation. The programs, conceived with the aim of reducing the number of children born with sickle cell disease, required that specific groups be screened for the trait rather than allowing them to participate voluntarily. In an overzealous and poorly-thought-out effort to eradicate the disease, some states passed laws requiring testing for diverse groups such as newborns, schoolchildren, applicants for marriage licenses, and prisoners. The program lacked most of the elements today recognized as crucial to an ethical genetic screening program. Specifically, many of the laws did not provide confidentiality of test results, free counseling services to those who tested positively, public education on genetic disease and the meaning of carrier status, guidelines

3. Steven R. Weisman, "No More Guarantees of a Son's Birth," *New York Times,* July 17, 1988.

to ensure that only the most accurate testing methods were used, or establishment of treatment facilities.[4] Current screening programs fulfill these criteria.

The predictable result was widespread misunderstanding, stigmatization, and resentment. From some of the legislation passed it was obvious that many lawmakers did not understand the distinction between carrying the sickle cell gene and having sickle cell disease. Certainly children could not understand the purpose and implications of the tests, and no provisions were made to ensure that they would receive adequate counseling when they grew up. Discrimination against carriers abounded. Some life insurance companies, for example, required that carriers of the sickle cell trait pay higher life insurance premiums, despite the fact that there was no evidence that they would live shorter lives than noncarriers. Some people recommended that demanding jobs such as police work, firefighting, and service in the armed forces be closed to carriers. Because at the time there was no way of diagnosing sickle cell disease in a fetus during pregnancy, the only way a couple who were both carriers could be certain that they would not have a child with the disease was to refrain from having children at all. Voices in the African-American community decried the racist implications of that alternative.

In light of the storm of protest that surrounded the early program, mandatory screening for sickle cell trait was discontinued. Ironically, in recent years it has been shown that giving antibiotics to an infant with sickle cell disease before signs of infection are evident can reduce the likelihood that the child will die in infancy or early childhood because of complications from infection. The concept of screening for sickle cell disease

4. Philip Reilly, "Genetic Screening Legislation," in Henry Harris and Kurt Hirschhorn, eds., *Advances in Human Genetics*, vol. 5 (New York: Plenum Publishing, 1975), pp. 319–376.

in newborns is gaining support, to offer children who are born with the disease the best opportunity for a healthy life.

The history of this ill-fated screening effort underscores the fact that a technology that can prevent genetic diseases does not exist in a vacuum. If it is to be used ethically, it must be considered within the confines of other technology and in light of political, cultural, social, economic, and educational factors. For example, in many hospitals termination of a pregnancy is currently allowed as late as the twenty-fourth week of gestation. Advances in neonatal medicine, however, may soon make it possible for babies born at that age to survive outside the mother's womb. Policies on selective abortion will need to be reevaluated. If a woman's access to abortion is restricted by new laws, her options for dealing prenatally with a severely handicapping condition will shrink—as they already have because of Medicaid's frequent failure to pay for abortions for poor women.

If prenatal screening is to be provided to the largest number of women in the most equitable manner, somehow the preexisting disparities in access to and use of early prenatal services will have to be addressed; for the later in her pregnancy that a woman obtains prenatal care, the fewer choices she has in dealing with any difficulties that arise. After the first trimester, for example, the mother cannot avail herself of chorionic villus sampling and, consequently, first trimester abortion of a severely damaged fetus is precluded.

Poverty and Prenatal Care

The American College of Obstetrics and Gynecology and the American Academy of Pediatrics recommend that visits for prenatal care begin as early in the first trimester of pregnancy as possible and be scheduled every four weeks until the twenty-eighth week, then every two to three weeks until the thirty-sixth week, and weekly thereafter. Yet according to the Institute of Medicine's Committee to Study Outreach for Prenatal Care, 18 percent of all infants born in the United States in 1985 were born to women who did not obtain prenatal care until the second trimester, 4 percent to women who obtained care only in the third trimester, and 1.7 percent to mothers who received no prenatal care at all. And only 68.2 percent of the total had what the committee deemed adequate care.

Certain socioeconomic factors are unambiguously linked to late and inadequate prenatal care. At a particular disadvantage are poor women, women whose health insurance is inadequate or nonexistent, and women in minority groups, particularly those who are African-American or Hispanic. Since about 33 percent of all births in the United States are to women with incomes less than 150 percent of the federal poverty line, the potential impact on the nation of inadequate prenatal care of these women is devastating. In 1980 about 65 percent of women with family incomes below 150 percent of the U.S. poverty level initiated care in the first trimester, compared to over 80 percent of those with higher incomes. Similarly, women with low incomes were three to four times more likely to receive late or no prenatal care than women with incomes above the 150 percent mark.

Interwoven with the problem of poverty is the fact that women often do not receive early prenatal care because they are ineligible for private health insurance or cannot afford to enroll in it, or what insurance they have does not include maternity care. By the mid-1980s more than 37 million Americans had no health insurance whatever from either private or public sources. About 14.6 million women of childbearing age have no insurance to cover maternity care, and 9.5 million of them have no health insurance at all, according to the Committee to Study Outreach for Prenatal Care.

The racial component of this problem cannot be overlooked,

and in fact appears to be worsening. Between 1969 and 1980, the percentage of women who obtained first-trimester prenatal care increased steadily. Then, especially for African-American women, the trend began to reverse itself, with an increase in the percentage of births to women who had obtained late or no prenatal care. In 1981, 8.8 percent of births to African-American women were in this category; by 1985, the figure was 10.3 percent. By contrast, among white women giving birth in 1985, 4.7 percent received late or no care. Hispanic mothers are substantially less likely than non-Hispanic white mothers to begin prenatal care early and are three times as likely to obtain late or no care. Moreover, Hispanic mothers as a group are more likely than non-Hispanic mothers to begin care late or not at all.[5]

George C. Cunningham oversees California's alpha-fetoprotein screening program for neural tube defects, which requires that doctors who see women between the fifteenth and nineteenth weeks of their pregnancies offer them this test. He notes that although 60 percent of women statewide choose to participate, only 20 percent of those seen at the Los Angeles County Clinic take advantage of the opportunity for alpha-fetoprotein screening. Large numbers of Hispanic women live in Los Angeles County, and Cunningham attributes their poor rate of participation to understaffing at the clinic, the long distances patients must often travel by public transportation to reach the clinic, the tendency to start care too late in the pregnancy, and their inability to speak English and consequent need for an interpreter.

Poor women fail to get appropriate prenatal care for many

5. Much of the preceding discussion is based on Sarah S. Brown, ed., *Prenatal Care: Reaching Mothers, Reaching Infants* (Washington, D.C.: National Academy Press, 1988); and Office of Technology Assessment, *Healthy Children: Investing in the Future* (Washington, D.C.: Government Printing Office, 1988).

other reasons. Some are so isolated from the mainstream of American society that they do not know how to obtain a doctor's services. As Floyd Malveaux of Johns Hopkins University said at a conference on the treatment of asthma, inner-city families sometimes live within blocks of the most sophisticated medical services in the world, yet are totally unaware of their existence.

Jennifer L. Howse of the March of Dimes, in a letter to the *New York Times* on September 19, 1988, described other "well-known" barriers: the shortage of doctors willing to accept Medicaid patients; overcrowded clinics, with long waits to be seen; impersonal care; inconvenient clinic locations and hours; a lack of bilingual staff and child-care services.

Among the solutions being tried in New York and several other states are the "fast-tracking" of patients through the Medicaid application process, the opening of satellite clinics to the large medical centers, the provision of transportation by van, on-site child care, and continuous supervision by the same physician throughout pregnancy. "There is scarcely a barrier to prenatal care that has not been overcome by at least one of the providers of maternity care," Howse noted in her letter. "The real challenge now is to promote and institutionalize these reforms . . . through changes in public health policy."

A number of governmental attempts have been made to equalize access to and encourage the use of prenatal services. The federal Office of Technology Assessment notes that publicly funded comprehensive prenatal care programs such as Maternity and Infant Care Projects, the Improved Child Health Project, and Improved Pregnancy Outcomes Projects, increase prenatal care among certain groups of poor women and adolescents. Through these programs more pregnant women get care earlier and more often.

In addition, the Omnibus Budget Reconciliation Act of 1986 (Public Law 99-509) gave states the option of expanding eligibility to pregnant women whose family incomes fall below the U.S. poverty level but above the states' Aid to Families with Dependent Children standards of need. Twenty-six states had elected to exercise that option by January 1, 1988.

Far more needs to be done. The Office of Technology Assessment describes the very process of enrolling in Medicaid as "a formidable barrier to the receipt of timely care."[6] States are allowed 45 days to process an application, but additional delays can be encountered when the applications are incomplete or other impediments arise. A General Accounting Office survey of poor women in 32 communities who gave birth found that about 6 percent of those who attempted to enroll for Medicaid experienced long delays in receiving notification of eligibility. The median time between application and determination of eligibility for these women was eight weeks.[7]

The Committee to Study Outreach for Prenatal Care believes that the severity of the problem warrants a fundamental overhaul of the way maternity care is delivered in this country. Specifically, it recommends that "the nation adopt as a new social norm the principle that all pregnant women—not only the affluent—should be provided access to prenatal, labor and delivery, and postpartum services appropriate to their need. Actions in all sectors of society, and clear leadership from the public sector especially, will be required for this principle to become a clear, explicitly, and widely shared value."[8]

The 1988 report of the congressionally mandated Commission to Prevent Infant Mortality (1988) also focuses vigorously on the need to reduce all barriers to prenatal care, including financial and bureaucratic ones.

6. Office of Technology Assessment, *Healthy Children*, p. 87.

7. General Accounting Office, *Prenatal Care: Medicaid Recipients and Uninsured Women Obtain Insufficient Care* (Washington, D.C.: Government Printing Office, 1987).

8. Brown, *Prenatal Care*, p. 13.

Inadequacy of Facilities

Although compassion dictates that this unfair access to early prenatal care, and hence prenatal screening, must be addressed, society must come to grips too with the fact that the development of prenatal diagnostic techniques has outpaced the health care system's ability to provide them. This problem is particularly relevant now that the cystic fibrosis gene has been found. Soon people with no family history of the disease will be able to undergo direct gene testing to determine whether they are carriers; it will also be possible to test newborn babies in this way.

Newborns can be tested for CF now by measuring the amount of trypsin (an enzyme secreted by the pancreas) in the blood. But only 85 percent of individuals with CF have a trypsin deficiency. Because the trypsin test misses 10 to 15 percent of the CF cases, it must be confirmed. The definitive test is the sweat test, so named because it detects the unusually high amount of sodium and chloride that people with cystic fibrosis produce in their sweat, making it salty. The test is painless and highly accurate, but it cannot be performed until the infant is two months old and may already show signs of the disease. (A baby younger than two months does not produce enough sweat for an accurate test.) When all the mutations in the cystic fibrosis gene are found and the DNA probes are perfected, direct gene testing will be more accurate than the trypsin test. It will be possible to perform the new test with confidence on the first day of life; and it will not require follow-up tests, thereby lessening parental anxiety.

At this point, scientists are still unclear about whether early identification and treatment of cystic fibrosis improves a child's health. A controlled clinical trial is currently under way at the Wisconsin Cystic Fibrosis Centers to evaluate the potential benefits of newborn screening for CF. One-half of the newborn

population is being screened at random, and newborns identified as having CF will be enrolled in a comprehensive evaluation and treatment program. Treatment options include pro-
phylactic vitamin and salt supplements, pancreatic enzyme
replacement therapy, antibiotics, and supportive respiratory
therapy to bolster their nutritional status. At the end of three
and a half years they will be compared with children who were
diagnosed by conventional means. After another three and a
half years, researchers hope to learn the effects of the early intervention. This type of analysis will be valuable in determining the benefits and risks of newborn screening for CF before it
is adopted on a routine basis. At the very least, recognition of
cystic fibrosis in a young baby would allow parents to know
they were carriers and act accordingly before they had other
children with CF.

One reason why it is important to know the advantages and
limitations of CF screening is that cystic fibrosis affects many
more people in this country than the other genetic diseases for
which mass screening programs have been undertaken: essen-
tially the entire population of Caucasian ancestry is at high
enough risk to warrant such an undertaking. The development
of screening tests for CF might well trigger the largest demand
for genetic screening and counseling ever experienced in this
country and necessitate a number of hard choices about who
would receive these services. Members of non-Caucasian races
also get CF, but at much lower rates, raising very difficult issues in this regard.

As noted by the President's Commission for the Study of
Ethical Problems, both the likely physical and psychological
benefits and the adverse effects on those screened, as well as the
relative costs and benefits to society, would need to be evalu-
ated during the determination of whom to screen and in what
setting. An extensive educational campaign would have to be
launched to inform the general public about CF. Unlike the

grass-roots efforts that are so much a part of the screening for Tay-Sachs disease, there are no subsets of the United States population that would have a vested interest in taking on this project.

To make an informed choice about whether or not to participate in screening, people at risk need to understand the nature and implications of cystic fibrosis. There are those, such as J. A. Dodge of Queen's University, Belfast, who find it unlikely that members of the general population would want to know their status as carriers. He attributes this to poor public education about genetics in general, and about CF in particular.[9]

One way to address this need is through a community-based program. Local resources would be used to inform people about the disease and about the test, which could then be made widely available. Some argue that the anxiety that might result from such a campaign could outweigh the benefits, as during the disastrous effort to screen for carriers of sickle cell disease. In addition, decisions would have to be made about whether to screen subgroups of the population, such as African-Americans (who have a much lower incidence of CF than the general population), children, and unmarried adults (who might want to know their carrier status before marriage).

An alternative means of applying the new technology would be to limit it to physicians' practices. Then pregnant women could be offered the carrier test, the partners of carriers could be tested, and prenatal diagnosis could be suggested for two-carrier couples. Such a system would involve 3 million pregnant women per year, the commission estimates. If we assume a carrier frequency of over 5 percent, about 165,000 carriers would be identified. If the partner of each carrier was then

9. J. A. Dodge, "Implications of the New Genetics for Screening for Cystic Fibrosis," *Lancet*, September 17, 1988, pp. 672–674.

screened, about 8,250 two-carrier couples would ultimately be found.

Unfortunately, the United States does not have the capacity to serve this volume of demand for diagnostic services. "The potential demand for CF screening is so large that even if a rather sizable portion of it does not materialize, an enormous demand for genetic counselors and other health care personnel and services could still be engendered," the commission noted.[10] Since ethical CF testing could not be offered without adequate support services such as trained counselors, public health personnel, public education, and community involvement, program objectives must either provide for the expansion of needed resources or limit screening initially in an equitable manner.

Neil Holtzman of Johns Hopkins University estimates that screening young women to determine whether their fetus had a chromosomal disorder or whether they themselves were carriers for just four serious disorders—cystic fibrosis, sickle cell disease, hemophilia, and Duchenne's muscular dystrophy—would entail more than 4 million tests a year. Approximately 46,000 of these would be positive and require follow-up. And this estimate includes only women seeking care during the first two months of their first pregnancy. Yet genetics centers currently serve 500,000 people each year at the most, Holtzman notes. Fewer than 1,400 professionals are currently certified by the American Board of Medical Genetics, and no more than 100 clinical geneticists and 75 genetic counselors with a master's degree are entering genetics each year. At this rate, with an attrition of approximately 25 per year, it will take at least a decade to double the number of geneticists.[11]

10. President's Commission, *Screening and Counseling,* p. 97.

11. Neil Holtzman, "Recombinant DNA Technology, Genetic Tests, and Public Policy," *American Journal of Human Genetics* 42 (April 1988): 624–632.

Because of this acute shortage of trained genetics profession-als, Holtzman anticipates that when DNA-based genetic tests become commercially available, they will frequently be offered by primary care physicians and others who have no specialized training in genetics. Yet a survey conducted in 1985 by the Education Committee of the American Society of Human Ge-netics identified 21 of 119 medical schools without a single formal course in genetics. [12] In addition, physicians who have been out of school for many years are unlikely ever to have been formally exposed to DNA-based genetic testing. Adding to the difficulty of conveying relevant information to prospective par-ents in a sensitive manner is the fact that the ethnic and cul-tural background of genetic counselors is often very different from those they are counseling.

TRANSPLANTING ORGANS

On a smaller scale, decisions related to prenatal diagnosis can engender conflict because they affect the mother, father, fetus, and health care provider differently. Take, for example, the matter of organ donation in the case of anencephalic babies.

These babies are born with most of their brain missing. The brain stem works fairly well, thereby allowing primitive func-tions such as breathing, but the infants have no higher brain activity and usually die within a week. As they deteriorate, they sporadically stop breathing, starving their organs of oxy-gen. By the time they die naturally, their organs are too dam-aged to use as transplants.

In October 1987 doctors at the Loma Linda University Med-ical Center in California transplanted the heart of an anence-phalic Canadian infant into another child with a hypoplastic

12. Vincent M. Riccardi and Roy D. Schmickel, "ASGH Activities Re-lated to Education: Human Genetics as a Component of Medical School Curricula," *American Journal of Human Genetics* 42 (April 1988): 639–643.

heart (one lacking the four normal chambers). After the operation the hospital received many offers of heart donations from couples who knew through prenatal diagnostic techniques that their infants would be born anencephalic and wanted to save the lives of other infants. As a result, the hospital began a short-lived program to use anencephalics as organ donors. Because of the ethical issues that arose, however, the hospital suspended the program nine months later. [13]

One of the major issues was the appropriateness of sustaining the anencephalic infants on life support systems for the benefit of those who would receive their organs. A person is considered brain dead only when the entire brain, including the brain stem, ceases functioning. Theoretically, then, an anencephalic baby is not brain dead, despite the fact that it is capable of only the most primitive activity. The hospital wanted neither to hasten the deaths of the infants, on the one hand, nor to keep them needlessly alive so that their organs would not deteriorate, on the other. The approach was to put the babies on respirators for one week, a time span in which 95 percent of anencephalic babies die. If the infants met the criteria for brain death within that time, their organs were made available for transplant. If not, the respirators were removed and the babies were allowed to die naturally with no subsequent use of the organs. For various reasons, none of the 12 infants managed this way was used as a donor of a major organ. One baby lived for two months, however. The emotional impact on the staff of maintaining infants in a vegetative state was one of the primary reasons for discontinuing the program.

Colleen Clements of the University of Rochester (New York) finds nothing innately wrong with intervening in the life of an anencephalic baby in a way that will not benefit that child, but rather another. In her monthly ethics column in the *Medical*

13. Peter Steinfels, "Infant Organ Plan Ends: Brief Lives, Large Questions," *New York Times*, September 18, 1988.

Post she wrote on February 16, 1988: "Organ donations can be made because of life support machines that really have no benefit for the patient, who is really dead in all but form. The family allows it because . . . it benefits others . . . If we're careful and respectful, people can be ethically used as means to an end or a purpose, if it's a purpose we all would share in as human beings. Philosophy, ethics, and medical ethics need to get back to the question of meaning and purpose in existence."

TESTING ERRORS

These types of issues would be difficult enough for prospective parents, their doctors, and society at large to resolve if the tests used for prenatal diagnosis were always accurate and reliable. In some cases, despite their best efforts, doctors cannot determine the outcome of a particular pregnancy. Sometimes a test wrongly indicates that a fetus has a particular condition when in fact it does not. Or the test will indicate that a fetus is free of a condition when it actually is not. Tests are also limited by the fact that they may identify a condition, but they cannot determine the impact of that condition on a person's life. Ultrasound, for example, may show the presence of a neural tube defect, but the physician may not be able to determine the severity of the defect and how it will affect the child's quality of life.

Errors that invalidate the results can also occur during testing. Sometimes through human error a blood sample is mislabeled during family RFLP studies. Results can be compromised if the doctor has misdiagnosed a condition. This can occasionally happen with cystic fibrosis, which resembles other pulmonary or digestive diseases. Genetic markers can be rendered useless through a rare process called recombination, in which the disease-causing gene is separated from its linked marker during chromosome replication.

Laboratory workers can make mistakes. Those who perform RFLP studies infrequently can confuse a regular polymorphism with a partial digest, a segment of DNA that results from incomplete cleavage of a DNA fragment. Although clinical laboratories must comply with state and, in some cases, federal laboratory practice standards, no states have yet established quality control procedures for tests involving recombinant DNA technologies.

Nor is genetic disease always the inevitable result of a single gene. In some families more than one faulty gene is needed to cause a condition that requires only a single gene in others. Environmental factors also influence whether a person with a genetic predisposition to a condition will actually develop it. And some people with positive test results suffer relatively minor manifestations of a condition that can incapacitate others.

WHO IS TO BE INFORMED?

Within the Family

Other troubling questions arise during prenatal screening. For example, clinicians may encounter sensitive information that could prove traumatic to one or more members of a family. Tests may show that a woman's husband or current partner is not the biological father of a particular child. This fact may become apparent when a couple comes in for counseling following the birth of a child with an autosomal-recessive disease, to assess their risk of having another child with the same condition. If the father proves not to be a carrier, he is almost certainly not the child's biological father. This information can also come to the fore during RFLP family studies.

At the 1988 annual meeting of the American College of Chest Physicians, Katherine Wood Klinger of Integrated Genetics in Framingham, Massachusetts, suggested that people be informed of this possibility when they express an interest in undergoing testing. Although this removes the onus from the genetic counselor of deciding what to do with any unwanted information, it can also provoke harmful conflict between husband and wife and discourage some women who would like genetic information from participating in the screening process.

Among the genetic counselors who took part in the 1987 multinational survey, 96 percent believed that protecting the mother's confidentiality overrode the need to disclose true paternity in such a case. Eighty-one percent said they would tell the mother in private and let her decide what to tell her husband; 13 percent would falsely tell the couple that they were both genetically responsible; and 2 percent would ascribe the child's disorder to a new mutation, a one-in-a-million occurrence. As the reason for their decisions, 58 percent cited preserving the family unit, 30 percent specified the mother's right to decide, and the remainder alluded to the mother's right to privacy. [14]

Although deliberately withholding information may prevent a conflict between husband and wife, it can create a plethora of new problems, as pointed out by the President's Commission for the Study of Ethical Problems. If both members of a couple erroneously believe they are carriers, they may forgo future pregnancies, try artificial insemination, or, if they conceive another child, needlessly incur the risk and expense of prenatal diagnosis.

A chromosomal abnormality of unknown meaning also presents problems. Telling the parents and testing them may cause anxiety, but not doing so may eventually cause more harm.

Outside Access to Test Results

The President's Commission concluded that genetic information should not be given to unrelated third parties, such as

14. Wertz and Fletcher, "Attitudes of Genetic Counselors."

insurers or employers, without the explicit and informed consent of the person screened or a surrogate for that person—unless serious harm would come to specifically identifiable individuals if the information were not disclosed. Yet in the survey of medical geneticists by Wertz and Fletcher, 58 percent of all respondents (63 percent if the United States is excluded), said they would tell the relatives of a patient with Huntington's disease that the patient had tested positively, even if that patient refused to permit disclosure. Twenty-four percent would go so far as to seek out and inform relatives even if they had not asked for the information. [15]

Ultimately, if the technology used for prenatal and other forms of genetic testing is to be used in an ethical fashion, participants must give their informed consent and be assured that the information will be used for their benefit. As Holtzman noted: "The protection of free choice depends on an educated citizenry aware of the purposes of genetic tests as well as their benefits, costs, and risks. This can be approached in a general way by improving public education but, more specifically, by assuring that genetic tests are only performed when the person offered the test has substantial understanding and will not be penalized as a result of either choice being made." [16]

What seem like simple tenets unfortunately can become so conflict laden that people turn to the courts to resolve their differences. Chapter 5 describes the legal issues involved in prenatal diagnosis.

15. Ibid.
16. Holtzman, "Recombinant DNA Technology," p. 629.

CHAPTER 5

Prenatal Diagnosis
and the Law

Citizens of the United States are guaranteed a number of basic rights by their Constitution. Particularly relevant to prenatal screening is the right to be free of governmental interference in deciding what will be done to people's bodies and how individuals will raise their children. Rights are conditional, however, and subject to interpretation by the courts. For example, although parents can decide in general what medical treatment their children will receive, the state can intervene if it feels that the choice threatens a child's life.

As the ability to screen for genetic diseases and diagnose them prenatally continues to evolve, so too does the legal framework that defines the rights and responsibilities of patients and parents, and the role of the health care professionals who serve them.

INFORMED CONSENT

In the United States competent adults must give their informed consent for any medical procedures they undergo. In practical terms this means that they may authorize or decline any diagnostic test or treatment and that their health care providers must give them the facts they need to make an informed decision. Specifically, the providers must tell them about the nature of their condition, the diagnostic and treatment measures that are available, and the alternatives possible for them—even if they must be referred to another provider.

In reference to genetic disease, patients must be told also the estimated risk of developing it and whether they are carriers for a particular recessive disorder. Genetic counseling must be based on an accurate diagnosis and should include an explanation of the implications for future and existing children of the family's genetic status. If they or their children have a genetic disease, patients should be told how the disease manifests itself and what can be done to treat or control it.

If a health care provider recommends a specific diagnostic procedure, such as amniocentesis or chorionic villus sampling, he or she must explain how it is carried out, what the benefits and risks are, and the implications of the test results. Health care professionals should be forthcoming about their level of experience and success rate with a particular procedure or treatment. An obstetrician who has done little chorionic villus sampling, for example, may not favor using it, although it would provide earlier prenatal diagnosis than amniocentesis. A patient may therefore want to consider consulting someone who has more experience with chorionic villus sampling so that she can not only obtain an early prenatal diagnosis, but have it done expertly and therefore more safely.

Another important aspect of informed consent is that patients have a right to receive the information in privacy and in terms they can understand. They should feel free to ask any questions that come to mind, and to obtain information in writing that they can study at their leisure before consenting to any part of a prenatal diagnostic work-up. They should not be timid about seeking another opinion if they do not understand fully the explanation given or desire additional assurance about a particular recommendation.

WRONGFUL BIRTH SUITS, WRONGFUL LIFE SUITS

Health care professionals who neglect to warn clients that they face an increased risk of passing a genetic disease to their off-spring, who misdiagnose a well-described hereditary disease, who do not explain what tests are available for evaluating this risk, and who fail to perform these tests competently and interpret the results, can be found legally liable. Two types of law suits can be brought against physicians under these circumstances: wrongful birth suits and wrongful life suits.

A wrongful birth suit is typically filed by a mother whose doctor did not tell her at a time when appropriate action could be taken that she was at risk of having a child with a genetic condition. As a result, she was robbed of the chance to make an informed decision about whether or not to carry through the pregnancy and bore a child with the condition. In a wrongful life suit, the case is brought on behalf of a child who would not have been born to experience the suffering caused by a genetic disease if the doctor had properly informed the parents that this was likely to happen.

The view of the courts has evolved over recent years from not awarding damages at all in wrongful birth suits to compensating parents for a range of expenses. The early approach in which no award was given stemmed from two factors: the desire to avoid giving the impression that an individual with a handicap was worthless, and the fact that before 1973 a woman carrying a baby with a genetic disease had no alternative to giving birth. The Supreme Court ruling in *Roe v. Wade* allowed women to choose abortion up to the twenty-fourth week of pregnancy.[1] In later cases parents won compensation for the medical expenses involved in raising a handicapped child. On

---

1. Roe v. Wade, 410 U.S. 113 (1973).

occasion they have received the costs normally associated with childrearing. Some courts have awarded damages extending into adulthood. Others have covered all the costs the person with the genetic disease is likely to incur throughout his or her lifetime.

The first wrongful birth case to reach a state supreme court was *Gleitman v. Cosgrove* in 1967. It involved a child born deaf and blind as the result of rubella suffered by his mother during pregnancy. The doctor had known that the baby might be impaired, but failed to tell the parents.[2] The New Jersey supreme court denied the parents and the child the right to sue on the grounds that it was impossible to compare an impaired life to no life at all. "A child need not be perfect to have a worthwhile life," the court wrote.

Ten years later the perspective had changed and the validity of wrongful birth suits was recognized. In *Becker v. Schwartz* the New York court upheld the right of parents to sue for medical expenses—but not for the emotional pain and suffering caused by rearing a defective child. The patient, Dolores Becker, had become pregnant at the age of thirty-seven. Her obstetrician, whom she had seen from the tenth week of pregnancy until the birth, did not tell her about the increased risk at her age of having a child with Down syndrome and the need for amniocentesis. She subsequently had a child with Down syndrome. The Beckers eventually gave up the child for adoption and settled out of court for the money they had previously spent on foster care.[3]

The case demonstrates what obstetrician Sherman Elias and attorney George Annas consider to be an excellent reason for allowing wrongful life suits, which courts are less prone to recognize than wrongful birth suits. As Elias and Annas point

2. Gleitman v. Cosgrove, 49 N.J. 22, 227 A.2d p. 693 (1967).
3. Becker v. Schwartz, 60 AD.2d 587, 400 NYS.2d 119 (1977); modified, 46 NY.2d 401, 386 NE.2d 807, 413 NYS.2d 895 (1978).

out, if the Beckers had won millions of dollars in their wrongful birth lawsuit and then given the child up for adoption, the
child would still not have been provided for. The alternative is
to allow children to bring their own lawsuits. "One can actually view wrongful life lawsuits as equalizers of a sort," they
argue. "At least in cases in which the child's parents are unable
to sue (e.g., because the statute of limitations has run out, or
because they have given their child up for adoption), this type
of lawsuit gives the handicapped child a chance to recover
money to pay for medical and custodial care, whereas in the
absence of such a remedy, the child would have no recourse
against anyone."[4]

The landmark wrongful life case involved a couple, the Turpins, whose first child was almost totally deaf but in infancy
was misdiagnosed by a specialist in hearing disorders as having
normal hearing. The Turpins then had a second child, a girl
named Joy, who had the same hereditary condition. The parents said that if they had known it was hereditary, they would
not have had another baby. The California supreme court
awarded medical expenses and special education expenses for
the hearing-impaired children. It refuted the implication that
a wrongful life suit devalues children born with birth defects.
It is "hard to see how an award of damages to a severely handicapped or suffering child would 'disavow' the value of life or in
any way suggest that the child is not entitled to the full measure of legal and nonlegal rights and privileges accorded to all
members of society," it wrote. The court also questioned the
assumption that the life of a severely impaired person is inher-
ently good, regardless of its quality. "Considering the short life
span of many of these children and their frequently very limited ability to perceive or enjoy the benefits of life, we cannot
assert with confidence that in every situation there would be a

4. Sherman Elias and George J. Annas, *Reproductive Genetics and the Law*
(Chicago: Year Book Medical Publishers, 1987), pp. 113–114.

societal consensus that life is preferable to never having been born at all."[5]

In another important wrongful life suit, a laboratory incorrectly reported that a couple, the Curlenders, were not carriers of Tay-Sachs disease. They subsequently had a child who did in fact have the disease. Because the laboratory had previously been told that their technical methods were inaccurate, the court awarded the child damages for medical expenses and pain and suffering based on her life expectancy of four years.[6]

COMPULSORY TREATMENT AND FETAL RIGHTS

An exception to the right to refuse medical intervention arises when the person who declines treatment places others at risk—someone with a contagious disease, for example. Under these circumstances the law permits mandatory vaccination and quarantine in the interest of public health. Some argue that genetic diseases are similar to contagious diseases in that they present a danger to other people, namely, offspring of the person known to be at risk of carrying a genetic disease. Extending their line of reasoning, they would compel a pregnant woman to undergo treatment against her will or mandate screening or prenatal diagnostic tests to avoid genetic diseases in future generations.

Geneticist and attorney Margery Shaw not only believes the comparison between contagious diseases and genetic diseases to be apt, she fervently advocates fetal protection. The state is well within its rights, she maintains, to compel parents to

5. Turpin v. Sortini, 31 Cal.3d 220, 643 P.2d 954, pp. 961–962, 963, 182 Cal. Rptr. 337 (1982).

6. Curlender v. Bio-Science Laboratories, 106 Cal. App.3d 811, 165 Cal. Rptr. 477 (1980).

"control their genes" and, if necessary, to abort a child with a severe genetic disease. In a landmark paper she notes: "Parents should be held accountable to their children if they knowingly and willfully choose to transmit deleterious genes or if the mother waives her right to an abortion if, after prenatal testing, a fetus is discovered to be seriously deformed or mentally defective. They have added to the burdens of the other family members, they have incurred a cost to society, and most importantly, they have caused needless suffering in their child."[7]

Her view stands in sharp contrast to U.S. Supreme Court decisions that people should have a "zone of privacy" in reproductive matters free from government intrusion, and that a woman's physical and psychological well-being transcend that of her fetus until the twenty-fourth week of pregnancy, after which the fetus may survive outside the womb. "The zone of reproductive privacy must be pierced in order for the state to gain control of fetal welfare," Shaw notes (p. 100), adding that the legal presumption that the mother's rights transcend those of the fetus should hold only if the fetus does not become a living child.

Others take strong exception to the notion that a pregnant woman can be forced against her will to undergo treatment on behalf of a fetus. Attorney Lori Andrews argues that the analogy to infectious disease breaks down, because a fetus cannot be treated without violating the mother's body. "Courts and legislatures should tread cautiously when considering mandatory screening, diagnostic, or treatment technologies involving pregnant women," she notes. "Not only do such forced services interfere with the woman's right to privacy to make reproductive decisions, they also have the potential for violating her bodily integrity in far greater ways than precedents

7. Margery W. Shaw, "Conditional Prospective Rights of the Fetus," *Journal of Legal Medicine* 5 (1984): 63–116; quotation on p. 111.

have allowed in the infectious disease situation. Compassion, communication, and attendance to the mother's needs—rather than a severe statute or cold court order—would seem to be the appropriate approach to give mothers a chance to provide needed medical care to their prospective child."[8]

In practice, women have been ordered to undergo treatment in only a handful of cases. In one particularly ironic instance a court ordered a pregnant woman, against her religious conviction, to undergo a cesarean section for the benefit of the fetus.[9] The patient, Jessie Mae Jefferson, notified the hospital that it was her belief that the Lord had taken care of her body and that whatever happened to the child was the Lord's will. Her doctor testified that there was a 99 percent certainty that her baby would not survive a normal delivery because the placenta covered the cervical opening. The hospital sought and obtained a court order to perform a cesarean section. Before the surgery could be performed, however, the baby was born normally.

We see here two of the major hazards of enforced treatment of pregnant women. First, it gives physicians extraordinary power over their female patients. Second, it denies women their constitutionally guaranteed right to autonomy and control over their bodies.

As shown by the case just described, physicians are not always right—and cannot be—despite the best of training and intention. Medical judgments are just that—judgments. If fetal rights are given total priority over those of pregnant women, and a doctor believes that a certain procedure is necessary or that the woman must act in a certain way to protect the fetus, a woman could find the intimate decisions about her

8. Lori B. Andrews, *Medical Genetics: A Legal Frontier* (Chicago: American Bar Foundation, 1987), pp. 234–235.

9. Jefferson v. Griffin Spaulding County Hospital, 247 GA, 86, 274 S.E.2d 457 (1981).

pregnancy being made by a judge, who may have different religious beliefs or values than she does.

Compulsory treatment "encourages an adversarial relationship between the obstetrician and the patient, and it gives the obstetrician a weapon to bully into submission any pregnant woman whom she or he views as irrational," say Elias and Annas. "Medical advice should remain advice: physicians are neither policemen nor seers." They also believe that it is unconstitutional to treat women differently when they are pregnant from when they are not. "To have a legal rule that there are no restrictions on a woman's decision to have an abortion, but if she elects childbirth instead, then the state will require her to surrender her basic rights of body integrity and privacy, creates a state-erected penalty on her exercise of her right to bear a child . . . Treating women as incubators while they are pregnant represses them and deprives them of their human dignity and autonomy, and so dehumanizes us all." [10]

Ellen Wright Clayton, of Vanderbilt University, has expressed concern about the fetal rights movement because it requires that women act in a way that men are not required to act. Parents are not compelled to undergo an invasive procedure such as donating bone marrow to their children, she notes.

> Yet this is precisely the type of intervention that many of the fetal therapy cases would impose upon pregnant women. Thus, there is a significant inconsistency between our society's views on the sanctity of the family as embodied in laws on child abuse and the approach taken by the proponents of forced fetal therapy . . .
>
> We must resist the temptation to intervene more deeply for the benefit of the unborn than we do for the children already among us . . . We seem to be moving toward a position that is

10. Elias and Annas, *Reproductive Genetics*, pp. 259–261.

doubly inconsistent—we protect children more before birth
than after, and we enjoin women to act on behalf of their unborn at the same time we withdraw the economic support that
would enable women to seek adequate prenatal care and diet. [11]

It would be ironic indeed to pass legislation forcing pregnant
women to undergo expensive, sophisticated medical treatment
against their will at a time when more and more of the United
States population lacks basic necessities such as housing and
food, as well as basic medical and dental services.

A recent example of the phenomenon addressed by Wright
Clayton took place in the District of Columbia. A twenty-nine-
year-old pregnant woman pleaded guilty to forging about
$700 worth of checks, a crime usually punished by a period of
probation. Because this woman used cocaine, which can cause
brain damage and retarded growth in a fetus, the judge sent
her to jail until her delivery date—to protect the unborn baby
from further exposure to the drug. [12]

Ensuring women's autonomy may result in harm to some
fetuses, but perhaps this is a necessary price to pay for freedom.
If a woman with phenylketonuria does not follow a low-
phenylalanine diet during pregnancy, she will almost certainly
have a severely retarded child. Yet it may be necessary to allow
this to happen in the small number of cases in which education
and support fail to change a woman's behavior. As Wright
Clayton notes, "It is important to distinguish what women, as
independent moral agents, may or even ought to choose to do,
from what women, as a class of citizens subject to potential
discrimination, may be required by law to do." [13]

11. Ellen Wright Clayton, "Women and Advances in Medical Technology: The Legal Issues," in *Biotechnology in Women's Health: Issues on the New
Frontier,* ed. Judith Rodin and Aila Collins (forthcoming).

12. Tamar Lewin, "When Courts Take Charge of the Unborn," *New York
Times,* January 9, 1989.

13. Wright Clayton, "Women and Advances."

MANDATORY VERSUS VOLUNTARY SCREENING

In a mandatory screening program everyone is obliged to participate. The only mandatory screening program presently under way in some states of this country involves testing newborns for metabolic diseases, primarily phenylketonuria. The test requires only that a small sample of blood be drawn; if the results are positive, treatment can be instituted before mental retardation sets in. Because some infants undoubtedly would be bypassed during the testing process if it were voluntary, this form of mandatory screening was approved by the National Academy of Sciences in 1975. It stands in stark contrast to the compulsory, short-lived screening for sickle cell disease carriers described in Chapter 4. The information gained in those tests provided no immediate benefit to the individuals screened, and no treatment was available to change their genetic status. Accordingly, the academy did not find the program appropriate. "Neither paternalistic nor public health nor public financial grounds seem to adequately support mandatory screening for other than reasons of medical intervention," it noted.[14] Screening for sickle cell disease carriers is now done successfully on a voluntary basis.

Maryland's program of screening for phenylketonuria is voluntary. Because of its strong educational component, cooperation in the effort is so great that it would take an estimated 500 years before a single case of phenylketonuria would be missed because of parental refusal to participate.

California's requirement that prospective mothers be informed about the availability of alpha-fetoprotein testing for neural tube defects holds promise and is in keeping with the

---

14. National Academy of Sciences, *Genetic Screening: Programs, Principles, and Research* (Washington, D.C.: National Academy Press, 1975), p. 189.

respect for autonomy assured by the Constitution. The impact of this law, and the provisions made to finance the testing, will be closely followed by many.

CONFIDENTIALITY

The information that is revealed during genetic counseling and the subsequent workup is sensitive and can be potentially damaging to the patient if it falls into the wrong hands. Generally speaking, physicians are ethically and legally bound to protect the confidentiality of their patients. Nevertheless, various third parties—law enforcement officials, public health authorities, relatives, employers, insurance companies, schools, lawyers—can request information about the patient, as we have seen.

A physician can release information only (1) when the patient has requested or agreed to its release; (2) when the law requires it; and (3) when the disclosure is necessary to protect a third party.

Lori Andrews urges that for their own protection patients be sure that the authorization to release information states specifically what information is to be released and to whom. Thus, if someone wants a relative told about the condition, the authorization should specify that individual and the information to be revealed. Andrews does not recommend signing a blanket authorization.

The problems and ethical issues that can arise when a person learns something about his or her genetic status that could harm another person (for example, a future child) but does not want to reveal this information to a spouse or blood relative were discussed in Chapter 4. The physician's legal role remains cloudy. "Apparently no courts have held that there is a duty to warn relatives of patients that they too may be at risk of genetic disorders," Andrews notes. She cautions that doctors who do so may be biting off more than they can chew. "Since the duty to disclose to relatives will be measured in part by the standard of care in the medical genetics community, exercising a right to disclose may ultimately set a standard creating a duty to disclose," she warns. [15] Physicians could find themselves in the position of having to track down all the close relatives of each of their unwilling patients.

In a sense this issue is theoretical. In most circumstances the person screened would have to supply the names of relatives before they could be contacted. The National Academy of Sciences cautions that relatives may very well not want this unsolicited information and may not be prepared to make good use of it: "Though relying on the consent of the initial patient screened does not guarantee that any relative contacted will welcome the genetic information, the possibility of benefit is at least increased when someone with personal knowledge of the relative has made the initial judgment that this information will be more useful than harmful." [16] Rather than take this burden on themselves, counselors would be better advised to establish guidelines with the patient at the beginning of the counseling process about who would be contacted and under what circumstances.

Another concern about confidentiality is that insurance companies may use information about people's genetic status against them. If private or public insurers are expected to pay claims for services, they have a right to access to the patient's medical records. On the other hand, consent can hardly be called voluntary if patients are threatened with nonpayment of their claims. Typically, they sign a blanket consent form allowing their insurance company access to all their medical records. Once the company has the information it may turn it over to a clearinghouse or data center such as the Medical Information

15. Andrews, *Medical Genetics,* pp. 197–198.
16. National Academy of Sciences, *Genetic Screening,* p. 187.

Bureau. Andrews warns that health care practitioners should not make disclosures to an insurance company other than the patient's, or for reasons other than to help the company decide whether to insure the patient or to pay a claim. "As various genetic markers are identified, policy issues will be raised regarding whether insurance companies should be allowed to use that information in making insurance decisions about individuals," she notes. "Now is the time for society to make judgments about what uses of personal genetic information are appropriate." [17]

17. Andrews, *Medical Genetics,* pp. 206, 19.

Conclusion

When we left Amy and Carl in the Introduction, they were reeling from the news that their son had Down syndrome. Indeed, during the first few months of Ethan's life his parents felt an odd mixture of sadness, fatigue, and joy. Ethan suffered none of the major heart defects common to children with Down syndrome, but he slept fitfully and had several ear infections. Amy extended her planned maternity leave from three months to six, so that she could tend him during the day. When Ethan was feeling well, he smiled a lot and stared with pleasure at the mobile of red and yellow elephants that hung over his crib.

Carl and Amy made an appointment with the genetic counselor and had karyotypes done on themselves. Both proved perfectly normal, leaving no explanation for Ethan's condition other than an accident of nature. The counselor outlined the risk of their having another child with Down syndrome and recommended that if Amy were to become pregnant again she should undergo chorionic villus sampling or amniocentesis.

As the end of Amy's leave approached, she found herself more and more reluctant to return to work full time and leave Ethan with a babysitter. She enrolled him in an infant-stimulation program the pediatrician had recommended. On Tuesday and Friday mornings they went to a medical center in the city and learned gentle exercises designed to improve Ethan's muscle tone.

It was at the center that Amy met Dottie and her adopted daughter, Mary Ellen. Over coffee one morning Amy learned their story. Dottie had worked as a secretary for many years before she met Hal, a firefighter. By the time they married it was too late for Dottie to have children, but she and Hal adopted Mary Ellen shortly after she was born. The fact that this couple chose a child with Down syndrome has brought a whole new perspective to Amy, and the presence of someone to talk with about the practical, day-to-day problems of living with a retarded child has been like a breath of fresh air.

Amy has always enjoyed working, and now her earnings are desperately needed. After long discussions with Carl and Dottie about good child care, and with her boss about her desire to work fewer hours in order to spend more time with her baby, Amy has been able to piece together a 30-hour work week from a combination of afternoons when she has arranged for child care with Dottie and evenings when Carl comes home early. Carl has taken on more of the shopping and meal planning and works on Saturday mornings while Amy minds Ethan. For the time being they are managing with this arrangement, but many details of the future remain cloudy. Carl and Amy still must decide whether they will have other children. With their decreased income and extra expenses, it seems unlikely, but they do know for sure that Amy will undergo prenatal diagnosis if she becomes pregnant. They need to decide what arrangements they will make for Ethan as he gets older. Right now he is a cuddly, loving child; but he will never be able to live independently, and this causes his parents much heartache.

This book was written for individuals like Amy and Carl and Dottie and Hal, who encounter genetic disease and prenatal diagnosis by choice or by chance. Even with the help of the most dedicated and patient physicians, parents must still make value judgments and tough ethical decisions that they can live with.

In the first few chapters we presented some of the basic scientific material that people can use as a springboard from which to elicit from their health care providers the information that they need. Although each case must be considered individually, certain generalities are possible about what constitutes appropriate prenatal screening.

Before a couple conceive a child they should discuss with their doctor how to maximize their chance for a healthy baby. This includes avoiding alcohol, drugs, medicines (except under the doctor's supervision), environmental toxins such as pesticides, and x-rays; following good nutritional and exercise practices; ascertaining immunity to German measles; determining their blood types; and so on. They should specifically discuss the possibility that they may carry a genetic disease. Certain people run this risk because of their ethnic background or other factors. If there is no specific risk of a genetic disease, at this writing the only genetic screening test during pregnancy that is routinely recommended is the serum alpha-fetoprotein test, which is done with a sample of the mother's blood taken during the second trimester. If the result of this test is higher than normal, the presence of a neural tube defect is suspected and must be explored. Ultrasound often shows that the fetus is older or younger than believed, and the parents may be reassured about the health of the fetus; but sometimes ultrasound shows that the fetus has the suspected defect. If the serum alpha-fetoprotein level is lower than normal, the fetus may have Down syndrome and the doctor will recommend the appropriate tests to evaluate the situation further. Amniocentesis can determine whether or not the fetus has a chromosomal abnormality.

If, because of family background, a couple is at higher than normal risk of having a child with a genetic disease, genetic counseling can help assess the chance of having children with that disease. Couples at risk should at least consider undergoing chorionic villus sampling early in the pregnancy or amniocentesis later, to determine whether the fetus is affected by a condition that cannot be determined before conception. Chorionic villus sampling or amniocentesis is also recommended for women over age thirty-five, who are more likely than their younger counterparts to have a child with a chromosomal abnormality. Ultrasound imaging is being used more and more frequently to assess potential structural abnormalities. And because research on prenatal testing is progressing very rapidly, the doctor or genetic counselor should be asked about the most recent available tests. For example, a new method for taking a sample of fetal blood from the umbilical cord is being tested.

The painful bottom line remains: finding out that a fetus has a severe genetic disease means that one must choose whether or not to continue the pregnancy, since treatment is rarely possible. Another distressing limitation of the new technologies is that they cannot always predict when a rare genetic disease will occur, and they cannot predict birth defects from most environmental agents or from unknown causes. No matter how much suffering prenatal diagnostic testing can prevent, it cannot guarantee everyone a healthy child.

We have also presented an overview of the ethical and legal issues emerging with the fast-moving technologies. Most people who have a genetic disease, or who love someone who does, will make a decision with the help of their doctor, just as they do in other areas of medicine. Only a very small number will turn to a lawyer to work out a dispute, or will find an unwanted third party involved in their private business.

Social, economic, and legal factors all enter into decisions about the availability of prenatal diagnostic technologies, as they compete with the many other elements of the nation's budget. The informed consumer is the best advocate for fair access to these services. Mounting pressures to restrict abortions, and the already existing constraints on the use of federal funds for this purpose, make safe abortions largely unavailable to poor women in many states, and therefore make prenatal diagnosis less useful.

Finally, although we have tried to make this book as practical as possible, it has no emotion or voice of its own. For most people who have a loved one with a genetic disease, the best source of help is a support group. There they can socialize with and learn from others in their situation. Many individuals in these groups make it a point to follow the latest scientific thinking about the disease in question; they may even be better informed than their doctors on this particular subject. They can also help with the everyday practical problems that arise when dealing with a genetic disease medically, personally, and socially. The more parents know, the better they can ensure that their child's health and emotional development are protected.

The Chamberlins had a 1-in-1,000 chance of having a child with Down syndrome so, according to accepted medical judgment, prenatal testing was not done. It is probable that as new tests such as the alpha-fetoprotein become more widely available, *all* pregnancies will be screened for this condition. But for Carl and Amy and many couples like them, the rarity of the problem afflicting their child is small consolation. For them, the frequency was 100 percent.

Society's attitudes toward handicapped persons have changed a great deal in recent years, however, reducing the barriers to social, employment, and other opportunities. There are legal requirements for education: handicapped children are no longer hidden away in institutions on the assumption that they would not know the difference.

This is not to say that families such as the Chamberlins have an easy time. Often medical care of handicapped children is very expensive and inadequately covered by insurance. Appropriate child care is hard to find and costly. The probable life-long dependency of their child on others is an emotional, as well as a financial, burden. Often pastoral or psychological counseling is needed; for if a marriage is not strong, it may break under the stress.

The impact of a handicapped child on siblings can be either beneficial or destructive. Brothers and sisters may feel cheated of parental attention as well as of material goods because the afflicted child requires so much. They may be embarrassed to bring friends home, or to go out with the handicapped child. But siblings may also learn compassion, responsibility, and altruism—and they may benefit greatly from the special love of the special child.

Even when a serious genetic disease runs in their family, the chance that a couple will have a healthy baby is at least one in two. We have seen that in the large majority of cases, prenatal testing assures prospective parents that their baby does not have the suspected problem. Many couples who otherwise might be afraid to try to have their own child can conceive knowing that the fetus can be tested and that they can choose to terminate the pregnancy if a serious problem exists. We hope that this choice will not be revoked. And we hope that this book will help prospective parents to make the choice that is the best possible one for them.

Appendix

Index

APPENDIX

Sources of Further Information

A number of nonprofit organizations stand ready to provide information to individuals with genetic diseases, their families, health care professionals, and other interested people. The list below is not intended to be complete; it is a starting point for obtaining additional information. The first three organizations concern themselves with genetic diseases in general. The others deal with a single disease or a single category of diseases.

A few publications are also included for those who wish to delve more deeply into some of the topics covered in this book.

Alliance of Genetic Support Groups, 38th and R Streets, NW, Washington, D.C. 20057. (202) 331-0942 / (800) 336-GENE. Joan O. Weiss, coordinator.

Provides information and support to people with genetic diseases and their families. Is a resource for community groups made up of people affected by the disease in question.

March of Dimes Birth Defects Foundation, 1275 Mamaroneck Avenue, White Plains, New York 10605. (914) 428-7100.

Aims to prevent birth defects, regardless of their origin, and is an excellent source of information about genetic diseases. Its *International Directory of Genetic Services* lists genetic service centers in the United States and in other countries. The address and phone number given above are for the national headquarters; for local offices, consult the white pages of your local phone directory.

National Center for Education in Maternal and Child Health, 38th and R Streets, NW, Washington, D.C. 20057. (202) 625-8400.

Provides information about all aspects of maternal and child health. Publishes a national directory, *Comprehensive Clinical Genetic Services Centers,* which lists treatment and evaluation centers by city and state.

Association for Retarded Citizens of the United States, 2501 Avenue J, Arlington, Texas 76006. (817) 640-0204.

National organization, with 1,300 state and local chapters. Provides detailed information about employment training and opportunities, guardianship and other legal matters, respite care, and financial assistance. A strong advocate for retarded citizens.

Cystic Fibrosis Foundation, 6931 Arlington Road, Bethesda, Maryland 20814. (800) FIGHT CF.

Huntington's Disease Society of America, 140 West 22nd Street, New York, New York 10011. (212) 242-1968.

National Association for Sickle Cell Disease, 4221 Wilshire Boulevard, Los Angeles, California 90010. (213) 936-7205.

National Down Syndrome Society, 141 Fifth Avenue, New York, New York 10010. (800) 221-4602.

National Hemophilia Foundation, Soho Building, 110 Greene Street, Suite 406, New York, New York 10012. (212) 219-8180.

National Tay-Sachs and Allied Diseases Association, 385 Elliot Street, Newton, Massachusetts 02164. (617) 964-5508.

Spina Bifida Association of America, 1700 Rockville Pike, Suite 540, Rockville, Maryland 20852. (800) 621-3141.

SUGGESTED READINGS

Emery, A. E. H. *Elements of Medical Genetics,* 6th ed. New York: Churchill Livingstone, 1983.

Goldfarb, L., M. J. Brotherson, J. A. Summers, and A. P. Turnbull. *Meeting the Challenge of Disability or Chronic Illness—A Family Guide.* Baltimore: Paul H. Brookes Publishing Co., 1986.

Grobstein, C. *Science and the Unborn: Choosing Human Futures.* New York: Basic Books, 1988.

Lynch, H. T., W. J. Kimberling, and K. M. Brennan. *International Directory of Genetic Services,* 8th ed. White Plains, New York: March of Dimes Birth Defects Foundation, July 1986.

National Institute of General Medical Sciences (Maya Pines). *The New Human Genetics: How Gene Splicing Helps Researchers Fight Inherited Disease.* NIH Publication 84-662. Bethesda, Maryland: U.S. Department of Health and Human Services, September 1984.

Nichols, Eve K. *Human Gene Therapy.* Cambridge, Massachusetts: Harvard University Press, 1988.

"Screening for Congenital Birth Defects." In *Guide to Clinical Preventive Services,* pp. 151–156. Report of the U.S. Preventive Services Task Force. Washington, D.C.: Office of Disease Prevention and Health Promotion, 1989.

Smith, D. W., and A. A. Wilson. *The Child with Down's Syndrome (Mongolism)—Causes, Characteristics and Acceptance: For Parents, Physicians and Persons Concerned with His Education and Care.* Philadelphia: W. B. Saunders, 1973.

University of Colorado Health Sciences Center. *Genetic Applications: A Health Perspective.* Lawrence, Kansas: Learner Managed Designs, 1988.

Weatherall, D. J. *The New Genetics and Clinical Practice,* 2nd ed. New York: Oxford University Press, 1985.

Weiss, J., J. E. Karkalitz, K. K. Bishop, and N. Paul, eds. *Genetic Support Groups: Volunteers and Professionals as Partners.* March of Dimes Birth Defects Foundation, Original Article series 22, no. 2, 1986.

Index